Doctors and Paintings

Insights and replenishment for health professionals

John Middleton

General Practitioner, Loughborough
Education Consultant,
LNR Deanery

Erica Middleton

Member of the Higher Education Academy
Associate Lecturer, The Open University
Tutor, University of Nottingham School of Education

Forewords by

Sir Liam Donaldson

and

Peter Wheeler

Radcliffe Publishing
Oxford • Seattle

Radcliffe Publishing Ltd
18 Marcham Road
Abingdon
Oxon OX14 1AA
United Kingdom

www.radcliffe-oxford.com
Electronic catalogue and worldwide online ordering facility.

Neither the publisher nor the authors accept liability for any injury or damage arising from this publication.

British Library Cataloguing in Publication Data

A catalogue record for this book is available from the British Library.

ISBN-10 1 84619 052 5
ISBN-13 978 1 84619 052 0

Typeset by Aarontype Limited, Easton, Bristol
Printed and bound by TJ International Ltd, Padstow, Cornwall

Dedicated to our children, Anthony and Rachael.

Contents

Foreword

Sir Liam Donaldson

Becoming and being a doctor is an enormous privilege. Doctors are afforded unrivalled access to the lives of their patients and they come into contact with all sorts of people: colourful and dull, warm and distant, vibrant and less so.

The unique window from which a doctor sees the world, intimately observing both the strengths and vulnerabilities of their fellow man, is a mixed blessing: doctoring brings joy but also discomfort.

Communication is the key to good doctoring and to ensuring not only a successful outcome for the patient but also a fulfilling career for the doctor. The importance of empathy is not to be underestimated. Art can help doctors to make sense of patients' lives and to adopt a range of perspectives in their work. It can be useful for understanding, communicating and coping. Art can help to build empathy.

In *Doctors and Paintings*, John and Erica Middleton guide the reader gently along the interface between art and medicine, in their own inimitable style. Reading this short book is no chore. Whether in search of an introduction to the world of art, or wishing to consider the role that the formal study of art might play in professional development, reading this book is likely to prove rewarding.

Turning these pages will help doctors to appreciate afresh the window through which they look upon the world.

Liam Donaldson
Chief Medical Officer
June 2006

Foreword

Professor Peter Wheeler

A recent article in the *Guardian* was punningly headlined 'Stressed workers enjoy art for heart's sake'. In the article, it was reported that after a 40-minute lunch break visit to the Guildhall Art Gallery, the stress levels of 28 City of London high fliers fell by 45%. The research was conducted by Dr Angela Clow, of the University of Westminster, who found 32% less cortisol in their saliva samples after their visit. It should be noted that among the favourite works in the Guildhall Collection are Victorian paintings by Constable, Millais, Rossetti, Leighton, Landseer and Poynton. These are relatively easy on the eye and the brain.

Shakespeare stated that 'Music soothes the savage breast', but he lived centuries before Igor Stravinsky, Arnold Schoenberg, John Cage, Charlie Mingus and Jimi Hendrix. Dr Clow's research applies this claim for music to the visual arts. Can painting soothe the savage breast? If I were a City of London high flier, I think that my savage breast could be soothed by spending 40 minutes looking at Constable's painting of 'Salisbury Cathedral from the Meadows', a favourite in the Guildhall Art Gallery. But if I were confronted with an exhibition of the 10 most headline-grabbing entries for the Turner Prize since its inception in 1984, would my stress level be reduced by 45% or would it have gone through the roof?

If, as Dr Clow's research suggests, the contemplation of art can be stress-reducing, so can the making of art. Christopher Southcombe, a painter now living in the Middle East, once worked as a Marine Society art tutor on Shell Oil Tankers (UK). In an article for the newspaper of the National Union of Marine Aviation and Shipping Transport, he wrote, 'Shell have an enviable safety record and part of Shell's philosophy is that men not machines cause accidents and that the possibility of accidents is increased when they are under stress . . .' The purpose of the Marine Society's art tutor scheme was to encourage seafarers to take up drawing and painting as 'a potentially very powerful antidote to stress'.

Dr Clow, psychoneuroimmunologist, and Christopher Southcombe, artist, make reasonable and believable claims for the direct therapeutic benefits of looking at and making art. Their work represents an extension of Art Therapy in the outside world of bankers and tankers. Art Therapy is normally associated with people in the inside world of psychiatric hospitals. Paradoxically, the art of psychiatric patients is sometimes called Outsider Art.

Since the intellectual liberation of the Renaissance, art and medical science have marched side by side in advancing the understanding of the human body.

Paintings of anatomists dissecting cadavers abound in the history of art. Many were included in a seminal exhibition that explored the long relationship between art and medical science. The exhibition was called 'Spectacular Bodies', subtitled 'The Art and Science of the Human Body from Leonardo to Now' and was shown at the Hayward Gallery, London from October 2000 to January 2001. The exhibition was divided into two parts. The first addressed the common interest of artists and medical practitioners in the human body. The second focused on the human face as a key to the understanding of character and temperament for artists, anthropologists and psychologists.

Since the Renaissance, it has been axiomatic that artists must 'acquire a mastery of the body as a functioning system of motion and emotion'. The Renaissance revived the idea, originating in Stoic philosophy, that 'man is the measure of all things'. This idea was enshrined within the belief that God's created order was designed for the understanding of the sentient human being, uniquely endowed with cognitive faculties including, most importantly, self-awareness and awareness of others. The Latin translation of a Greek inscription on the Temple of Apollo at Delphi is 'nosce te ipsum', in English: 'know thyself'.

'Know thyself' is very much the leitmotif of this unique book, jointly written by a dedicated general practitioner and an equally dedicated painter. 'In the western cultural tradition, as in much of the art originating from other cultures, the representation of the human form has played a central role in the quest to deal with the great issues of birth, life, humanity and death in relation to the transcendent reality of the divine.' This quotation from the introduction to the catalogue for 'Spectacular Bodies' chimes with the statement in the introduction to *Doctors and Paintings* that 'The issues that concern patients, their doctors and also artists include sex, death, power, money and spiritual belief'.

The book is written in form of a discourse between three GPs with discursive interjections from Liam and Donald. It is close to being the text for a play. The basis of the discourse is that artists deal through their work with the big issues of the human condition: identity, gender, sexuality, success, failure, health, illness, ageing and finally, mortality, in the context of spiritual belief or the lack of it. Every working day, doctors have to help their patients deal with the same issues. The thesis is that by understanding how the Arts address the 'great issues', doctors can develop greater awareness of these issues in relation to their own lives and, through greater self-awareness, a greater capacity for empathy with their patients and their problems.

Empathy is the capacity to experience vicariously the feelings, desires and thoughts of others, the ability to 'put oneself into another's shoes'. It is a translation of the German word 'Einfuhlung', meaning 'feeling in' in the sense of feeling oneself into the inner life of another person, into the forms of inanimate objects and into the form and content of works of art.

'Einfuhling' was a theory, from nineteenth-century German philosophy, that attempted to explain how we are affected by works of art. In today's world, the shared aim of professional curators, critics, art historians and educators is to help the art public to arrive at a critical understanding of art. Art may be understood from a variety of critical positions: modernist, postmodernist,

Marxist, psychoanalytical, feminist or multiculturalist. From wherever the critic comes, the practice of critical understanding involves three closely interwoven and interdependent elements: description, interpretation and evaluation. Before the meaning of a work can be deduced, speculated upon or wondered at, it is necessary to know what is in a work of art that is visible and can be described. All works of art have subject matter or content, they have formal characteristics and they provide evidence of the artist's use of and response to media, materials and technical processes. Subject matter, form and medium are all describable.

An exercise to make art students look more than superficially at a work of art requires them to write down 20 questions about subject matter, form and medium, to which they would like an answer from the artist, whether dead or alive. From the process of interrogating a work of art in this way, it is possible to come up with an inventory of describable information. To this, external information can be added, about the artist and the historical context in which the work was made.

In looking closely at a work of art, questions inevitably arise about what meaning or message is contained within it. In most critical writing or discussion about art, description dissolves almost imperceptibly into interpretation. Description addresses what is in the work, whilst interpretation addresses what the work is about. All works of art have content and all works of art have 'aboutness'. The content of a seventeenth-century Dutch still life may be a skull, a book and a candle. These are not neutral objects, but symbols. The painting is about the transitory nature of human existence, in which the iconographical theme is 'Vanitas'. Iconology is the word for the interpretation of meaning in art through symbols and symbolic traditions. It is an analytical method applied mainly to art of the more distant past, particularly where little or nothing is known about the artist. Critical interpretations of most modern and contemporary art rely heavily on external information about the artist and the context for production. Interpretations are rhetorical arguments and may be based on the critical position from which a critic writes, creating debate around the meaning and the value of a work of art.

As description dissolves into interpretation, so interpretation dissolves into judgement or evaluation. Interpretation addresses 'aboutness'; judgement addresses quality. Interpretation is based on knowledge presented as evidence. Judgement is based on criteria presented as evidence. Interpretation and judgement are rhetorical, attempt to be persuasive, and will succeed or fail in the attempt. Judgement is applied to most contemporary art as soon as it is put in the public domain. Some critics judge the art of their time to be bad art or even not art according to their criteria. History frequently overturns their judgement. History applies the 'test of time' as a quality assurance guarantor. On the basis of their lengthy discussions and visits to museums and galleries, Liam and Donald should be encouraged to play Art History Fantasy Football and to debate the make-up of an all-time greatest world team of 11 artists (and some reserves) from all ages and all places. There will need to be selection criteria, which the doctors of the discourse should specify, now that they have knowledge of artists who have dealt, in their art and their lives, with the big issues.

This foreword ends with the proposition that there may be a parallel between what is involved in the critical understanding of art and the diagnostic practice of the general practitioner. It seems to me that the descriptive phase of critical understanding corresponds with the initial interaction between the patient and the GP. In answering the GP's opening question 'What seems to be the problem?', the patient describes his or her symptoms, which are then investigated both verbally and through physical examination. This phase for both the art critic and the GP may be characterised as 'getting the picture'.

Interpretation corresponds with diagnosis, both of which are based on knowledge and experience and also in some measure, intuition and imagination, applied to the visible, describable content of a work of art and to the symptoms and signs of a patient. Just as there can be multiple interpretations of a work of art, a patient can seek a second opinion. In the case of multiple critical interpretations some may be more convincing than others, depending on the predisposition and the knowledge of the critic's reader. In the case of medical diagnosis, a patient may be more convinced by one of two or more opinions, but one is more likely to be right than others. Interpretation and diagnosis are revelatory and demonstrate the capacity to 'understand the picture'.

Judgement proceeds from understanding. The critic judges a work to be good or bad, interesting or not, again based on knowledge, experience and personal criteria. The critic makes value judgements. Based on diagnosis, the GP uses judgement to help the patient to decide what is best for them, for example referral to a consultant.

Doctors today work under enormous pressure. It must often seem that reception areas, in surgeries and health centres, are heaving with people waiting to unload their problems on their GPs. Great art provides insights into the human condition. If through a systematic engagement with art and literature as an extension of their medical practice, GPs can apply those insights to themselves (know thyself), they can equally apply them when dealing with patients. Doctors and patients are people, subjects. Intersubjectivity is perhaps a better word than empathy to define what this book seeks to promote, the capacity of the doctor to enter into and inhabit the patient's subjectivity.

Peter Wheeler
Dean, College of Fine Arts
University of Sharjah
United Arab Emirates
June 2006

About the authors

John has been a GP in the same practice since 1978 and a trainer since 1980. Presently, he is involved in supporting professional development for experienced trainers. He has written widely in medical journals and has a body of published research in the field of communication. Many of the ideas are brought together in his book: *The Team Guide to Communication*. Apart from this, there are two unpublished novels in the loft, an opera, an oratorio and a symphony. Extracts from the opera have recently been performed, much to the bemusement of some of the patients who thought they knew him. He is often to be seen running with the dog, at the crack of dawn or before. However, it has to be said that he can't paint for toffee.

Erica has a foot in both camps – painting and art history. Each informs the other. She teaches both art history and practical courses at undergraduate level for the Open University and the University of Nottingham. As a painter, she has researched on a practical level the nature of traditional materials such as genuine pigments, paint binders and gilding, in order to facilitate an old master look for contemporary themes. Her work can be viewed at www.minigallery. co.uk/Erica_Middleton. She has recently exhibited at the Lorenzo Lotto Academy in Mirano, Venice and is on the committee of Loughborough *Artspace* www. artspace-lboro.co.uk. And she does *everything* in the house and garden . . .

Acknowledgements

Our thanks go to Susan West MA (Oxon) PhD for the time spent with Photoshop making the illustrations suitable for publication.

Thanks are also due to the following owners of paintings who have agreed to them being published: Professor Peter Wheeler; Mr & Mrs S Kelly; and Mr & Mrs B Schou.

Erica's paintings

'What an artist is trying to do for people is to bring them closer to something, because art is about sharing: you wouldn't be an artist unless you wanted to share an experience, a thought. I am constantly preoccupied with how to remove distance so that we can all come closer together, so that we can all begin to sense that we are the same, we are one'.

David Hockney (2004) *Hockney's Pictures*. Thames & Hudson, London.

Introduction

This book is the culmination of a 27-year conversation about art in relation to medicine between the authors, who have just celebrated their silver wedding anniversary. Components of the book, whilst being written by one, have therefore been deeply influenced by the other over this time. Furthermore, there have been inputs by the other at every stage of the writing, so that the entire work is an integration of the two rather than 'his 'n' her' parts. Having said this, generally speaking, Erica is responsible for the arty bits and John is responsible for the medical bits. We decided to use a ubiquitous first person, whichever of us was the main writer at the time, in the hope that it would be less confusing.

Donald and Liam first appeared in John's previous book, *The Team Guide to Communication*, where they were described variously by reviewers as being like a Greek chorus or something out of the Muppet Show. They can usually be relied on to expose faulty logic or plain pomposity, but also afford a bird's-eye view of the action. This concerns the interaction of the three doctor characters (two of them also from the *Team Guide*), their patients and the art tutor. All of these characters are figments of the fevered imagination. Any resemblance they may bear to anyone you know, or may have heard of, is purely accidental. Moreover, the views that any of them express should not be taken to represent those of the authors.

You might approach the book in a variety of ways, depending on who you are and what you want. If it's the bottom line you are after – there is a summary of the argument at the beginning of each chapter. This argument can be followed with reference to Erica's paintings, reproduced here. For those who want to engage more deeply with the world of painting, there are plentiful references to other artists and their work interwoven with the text. Where possible, these are linked to websites so that you can view the images on-line, perhaps with the book on your knee. Unfortunately, precise web-addresses are subject to change, but search engines can usually help you to locate the pictures you want. For this reason, many of the references are in the form of key words which the authors have verified on Google – www.google.co.uk. In addition, there is a list of references to literature at the end of each chapter.

However, you may notice that the book begins to function almost as a novel, because the characters develop (or at least reveal themselves) as the book unfolds. Whilst you are welcome to dip in and out as you please, the experience may perhaps be richer if you are aware of what has gone before. Nevertheless, we have repeated some of the stories about the paintings that appear in more than one chapter to accommodate readers who prefer to take it in a different order.

There are two threads that run through the book: doctors primarily as people, and patients primarily as people. Each have their own respective (and often private) fears, worries and agendas. These individuals are artificially thrown together into an ongoing partnership in flux. When clinical medicine seems inadequate in addressing the interaction, where else can doctors turn? One answer might be art. The focus here is on painting, because this is Erica's long-term medium.

The issues that concern patients, their doctors and also artists include sex, death, power, money and spiritual belief. Once you engage with paintings at more than a superficial level, it is impossible to duck them. Being present as another human being means sharing these concerns. A short work can only scratch the surface, but some of the scratches might be deep. Humour is one way of coping, but none of it is intended to be malicious. At least we made each other laugh.

CHAPTER 1

Liam and Donald go to Tate Modern

'Here we are at last – in the Turbine hall,' says Liam, 'Don't you think it's like a cathedral?'

'Wish they'd left the turbines,' says Donald.

'Well, at least I've finally dragged you here,' says Liam.

'You promised me football,' says Donald suspiciously.

'Later, later,' says Liam, patting the tickets in his back pocket, 'but first things first.'

'Bribery will get you anywhere,' says Donald, 'but I still don't understand why you're doing this.'

'It's an experiment, Mr Spock – to see whether someone with a mind like yours can connect with painting.'

'It is not logical, Captain.'

'People are not always logical, Spock. They have intuitions and feelings; that's where art comes in.'

'I thought doctors were supposed to suppress their feelings – keep them for weekends,' says Donald.

'Very droll,' says Liam, 'but you're not a doctor, so listen up – you might learn something.'

'The programme is busy,' says Donald; 'press any key to continue.'

'I know you're in there somewhere,' says Liam, 'but, talking of cathedrals, you really have to see the Rothko room.'

The Rothko room is situated within the *Landscape/Matter/Environment* section of the thematically organised Tate Modern. It is a compact space, with reduced light – both factors being in accordance with the artist's wishes. It comprises seven huge maroon and black/grey abstracts which feature variations on rectangular compositions with soft focus edges. The whole, as an expressive environment, was influenced by Michelangelo's Laurentian Library in Florence where blind windows contributed to an oppressive atmosphere.

> These canvases were the result of a commission in the 1950s for the Four Seasons Restaurant in the Seagram Building on Park Avenue, New York. Having produced the canvases Rothko felt their brooding character to be inappropriate for the setting of a fashionable restaurant where deep contemplation would be impossible. So he withdrew the commission and presented the Seagram Murals to the Tate, referencing his deep debt to JMW Turner.

'Not much to this lot,' says Donald.
'Why do you say that?' says Liam.
'Well they're just like big daubs. I could do it. Just give me a few cans of emulsion!'
'But don't you think that they have a monumental feel?'
'Monumental?'
'Yes – like Stonehenge.'
'Don't know about Stonehenge, but they are a bit like goalposts!'
'Trust you to bring football into it!'
'Ssh!,' says Donald. 'People are looking at us.'
'All right,' says Liam. 'I'll be quiet.'

Donald gazes around the room aimlessly for a while.

'Help!' says Donald.
'What?'
'I can't get much out of this. Where should I stand?'
'About eighteen inches away,' says Liam.

(This is the distance Rothko himself recommended, though different 'readings' are facilitated through viewing from different distances.)

Donald approaches one of the canvases very closely and takes up a solid stance, with a furrowed brow. After a few minutes he tries another canvas, then another.

'Don't like these paintings,' says Donald. 'Get me out of here!'
'Don't like?' says Liam. 'Why not?'
'Gives me the "willies",' says Donald. 'Makes me feel depressed.'
'Yay!' says Liam.
'What do you mean 'Yay'?'
'It's a reaction! Means you feel something, Mr Spock!'
'I don't see why you're so pleased. I didn't come here to be made to feel depressed. Is that what's in store for the doctors? I should think they need cheering up after a hard week's work.'
'Stay with it for a moment, please,' says Liam. 'Why do they make you feel like that?'
'It's all that black space – and those goalposts crowding in on you,' says Donald.
'I think you made me stand too close. Is there somewhere we can get a coffee?'

They proceed in search of coffee, but drop into the shop en route. This is the largest book-shop of any art gallery in Britain. It stocks over 10,000 different book titles and 70 products are made exclusively for the Tate. These range from T-shirts and posters to a very comprehensive academic art history section. Liam and Donald head for the latter, still reeling from Rothko.

'Doesn't Rothko make you feel depressed, too?' says Donald.

'As a matter of fact, no.'

'What about all that nothingness?'

'For me, it's infinite space,' says Liam.

'Yes Captain, the final frontier,' says Donald, 'but look – I don't enjoy feeling stupid about art. Can't you find me a manual here which explains everything?'

'Let me buy you a present,' says Liam. 'Its called *Painting and Tears* by James Elkins. The first chapter is all about Rothko.'

'Sounds a bundle of laughs,' says Donald, 'but I'll give it a try. Now can we lighten up a bit?'

'Okay,' says Liam. 'Talk to me about football.'

'Never thought you'd ask. What do you want to know?'

'Well you, Mr Spock, who is supposed to be so unartistic, often talk about beautiful goals. That interests me.'

'I am surprised! Never thought you had the slightest interest in football!'

'Why are they beautiful, Donald?'

'It's the movement . . . the patterns leading up to the goal; the speed and energy, I suppose.'

'Like ballet?'

'Not a bit like that!'

'Like painting, then?'

'How so?'

'The movement of the brush; the patterns of the marks; and also the speed and energy of the brush strokes.'

'That's as may be, but I'll tell you what isn't at all beautiful.'

'Go on.'

'A goal scored against your team, by the opposition!'

'What you mean is that beauty is in the eye of the beholder,' says Liam.

CHAPTER 2

Doctors for the people

Doctors must deal with people in their social context as well as with their illnesses. To engage effectively, person to person, demands a high degree of self-awareness on the part of the doctor.

Once upon a time, Dr Strait had a rather taxing surgery. His first patient was 79-year-old Mr Choleric, with a systolic blood pressure of 190. He knew it would take a long time and it did. The trouble was that you couldn't afford to have many long appointments, if you were obliged to see anyone who insisted on coming the same day. He didn't see how someone like old Choleric could be managed by telephone triage.

That systolic blood pressure had stuck obstinately around the 190 mark for the last seven or eight months. Mr Choleric was on four different anti-hypertensive drugs and he did not like the side-effects.

'Can't see much painting in this,' says Donald.
'Just you wait and see!' says Liam.

Choleric was always difficult, perhaps always had been. He still wore a dark suit and a tie to his appointments with the doctor, though his shirt was often slightly stained and he no longer shaved very efficiently.

'I'm thinking Rembrandt late self-portraits,' says Liam.
'You don't mean those brown depressing things?' says Donald.
'I'll explain later,' says Liam (see Chapter 5).

Dr Strait was running out of options. He'd tried explaining the pros and cons, with evidence for the various alternatives (and boy, did that take a long time!), but old Choleric just kept saying 'you're the doctor'. Infuriating when you don't have the answers. He kept seeing himself (and didn't want to), not so many years down the line, facing similar dilemmas. Tied to tiresome routines of taking cocktails of drugs. Made miserable by the side-effects. Surely life was for living? The quality was the important thing. But then, what if he had a stroke and didn't die? Perhaps better to suffer a moderate degree of side-effects than risk such a fate? Not that anyone could tell you for sure; statistics don't work for individuals – only for populations. And was the science to be trusted? Was it all part of a marketing exercise by the multinational corporations?

'He's paranoid, isn't he?' says Donald.
'But listen!' says Liam. 'Those thoughts he's having might help him to understand the patient a bit more.'
'You mean they're in the same boat?' says Donald.
'Well, they're both human beings, at any rate.' Says Liam. ' They are both on a one-way ticket and getting nearer the end of the line.'
'Thanks for that cheerful thought!' says Donald. 'How does it help exactly?'
'It's the human condition,' says Liam. 'Perhaps we can get some help from the artists?'
'I wish I shared your confidence,' says Donald. 'Seems to me that they need help sorting themselves out, never mind the rest of humanity. Anyway, this guy Choleric probably just needs his blood pressure treating properly. If Strait doesn't know enough about it, he should send him to someone who does!'
'Don't you think he hasn't thought of that already?' says Liam. 'This man is already on four different drugs for blood pressure, and he's very likely been to see a specialist. His arteries are probably stiff and that's why it's difficult to make any impression on the blood pressure, not without getting lots of side-effects.'
'Didn't know you were a professor of medicine as well!' says Donald.
'It's all on the internet,' says Liam, 'but you can't really think that this is just a physical problem, can you?'
'Yeah, yeah – physical, social and psychological – heard it all before!' says Donald.
'And spiritual,' says Liam.
'And fairies at the bottom of the garden!' says Donald.

Feeling overwhelmed and exhausted, Dr Strait decided to refer Mr Choleric back to the specialist. Not that this would solve the problem. He knew very well that the appointment would take a few months, and that Choleric would be back to see him many times before that. Also he knew that the specialist would see his patient only once, and discharge him before waiting to see whether any new intervention had worked. He would probably do the same himself in that position. But at least he would have shared the therapeutic dilemma with someone else. The feeling of being alone was perhaps made slightly less.

Later that day, 73-year-old Mr Tidy came back to see Dr Shorts. It was his twentieth visit to the doctor that year, and it was only September. As always, he was very apologetic about taking up the doctor's time. As usual, he gave a careful account of his bowel action since his last visit. It was always a bit variable and Mr Tidy had helpfully made notes on the variations in his diet that might or might not have contributed to the situation.

Dr Shorts had already referred Mr Tidy to the surgeon. On a previous occasion they had found a polyp in the colon, but it had turned out to be benign. Despite reassurance from the specialist, Mr Tidy continued to keep his 'diary' of bowel activity and to report it regularly to his GP. Dr Shorts had come to see his role as one of protecting his patient from unnecessary further investigation, and also saving expensive resources.

At first sight it wasn't too difficult. Short-term changes in bowel habit don't justify referral for investigation. The problem was that each visit to the GP added another week or two to the duration of symptoms; and what exactly constituted a change in bowel habit anyway? Mr Tidy's bowel habit was *always* variable, so perhaps it was normal for him?

Usually Dr Shorts examined Mr Tidy's abdomen. Sometimes he organised blood tests and stool examinations. Occasionally he did a rectal examination, but didn't find anything. The patient always seemed to go away satisfied, though he kept returning at short intervals. When Dr Shorts had referred him to the specialist last time, it was because he (the doctor) had reached the limit of his anxiety. Eventually, thought Shorts, I am going to miss something important with this man – just because he gives me too much information!

A few days later, Dr Shorts had the opportunity to bring the case up with his colleague: 'What does he want from me?' he asked, over coffee.

'He just wants to make sure he won't die,' chuckled Dr Strait.
'Surely he doesn't think that seeing me for a check-up every few weeks will make him immortal?'
'Why don't you ask him?' said Dr Strait.

'Rothko, this time,' says Liam.
'The goal posts guy? Don't tell me – you'll explain later!' says Donald.
'I will – but listen!' says Liam. 'You were just now sneering about the relevance of the spiritual dimension. Here is a man who is scared of death. Why? What does he believe, or not believe in?'
'Dunno,' says Donald; 'nobody's asked him. Do you think that's an appropriate job for a doctor?'
'It's a good question,' says Liam, 'but you will admit that there's more to being a doctor than just managing blood pressure.'

'Anyway,' said Dr Strait, '*my* patient *knows* he's going to die; he's just unhappy about the process leading up to it.'
'You mean ageing?' said Dr Shorts.
'Means more to me than you, I guess,' said Dr Strait, fingering his grey whiskers.

Elsewhere in the building, Dr Susan was into the sixteenth minute of her consultation with 47-year-old Mrs Liszt. This week it was abdominal pain, just when she thought that all *that* had been dealt with.

'Oh dear!' said Dr Susan, as she listened to all the details, 'It must be terrible for you.'
(She thought: more tests and maybe another referral to add to her collection? She must be unhappy, but she won't have it that the symptoms might be psychological. Just when I think that we could be getting somewhere with a problem, she tries a different tack. She seems to know how to trigger the guidelines for urgent

referrals, or at least to make me worry about them. I feel that I'm making no progress with her, and she's not the only one.)

Dr Susan was going to be late again. Then she had to do the shopping and cook the dinner. Her surgeries seemed to be full of people with anxiety and depression, and multiple symptoms. When she went on holiday, they waited for her to come back. She needed a holiday right now; she was so tired. What she didn't need was the rush of patients, before and after the holiday, all insisting on seeing *her*. It was good to know that she was popular with the patients. She supposed that it was a measure of success – of doing a good job, but sometimes she had the feeling that she was everyone's mother – a universal recipient of problems!

'Don't tell me this time!' says Donald, 'It's Munch, isn't it?'
'You mean The Scream?' says Liam. 'Who's screaming – the patient?'
'No,' says Donald, 'the doctor!'

Later that evening, Dr Shorts put his feet up with a warm drink and his personal learning plan (Dr Susan was still doing homework with her children, and Dr Strait was having a visit from his financial adviser about pensions and inheritance tax avoidance). He opened his well-thumbed copy of *The Team Guide to Communication*, which he kept at the ready for trainer re-approval visits. It fell open naturally at the diagram of the *face model* (see Figure 2.1).

'Remind me why it's called the face model,' says Donald.
'Two eyes, a nose and a mouth,' replies Liam, at once
'Doh!' says Donald.
'It's easy,' says Liam. 'The two eyes are the **agendas** *– those of the patient and the*
doctor. The mouth is what comes out of the interaction – the **negotiated plan.**'
'And the nose?'
'That's the bit that connects everything – **skills.**'
'I think I might prefer the Art!' says Donald.

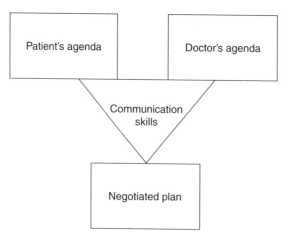

Figure 2.1   The 'Face' Model

The patient's agenda, thought Dr Shorts; that was the key to everything, according to Middleton anyway.[1] Why was it so important? After all, the doctor had plenty of important things on his agenda, too – clinical indicators, for example. Quality of care was in the best interest of the patient, wasn't it? Ah, but then all the doctors' efforts were wasted if the patient was going to take no notice. They had to feel that their agenda was being addressed and that the plan was relevant to their needs.

But what about Mr Tidy? What was his agenda exactly? What if the agenda was too difficult to handle? What if he didn't have any answers? Was there some kind of existence after death and, if so, what would it be like? If not, did it matter, since he wouldn't know anything about it? Doctors were supposed to have it all worked out – dying and bereavement. What was the expression they had used at medical school: 'being *comfortable* with your own mortality'? Dr Shorts found it slightly disturbing to be faced with the same questions he thought he had resolved a long time ago. If indeed it was a spiritual issue behind Mr Tidy's frequent consultations, was it right for a doctor to confront it, and did he really want to?

Dr Strait poured himself another measure of Lagavulin. Surprise, surprise – the Chancellor had covered all the loopholes that mattered. If you could know how long you were going to last, and in what sort of condition, it would be easier to make plans. He didn't mind giving money to his grandchildren, so long as he had enough left for his own needs. But how much could he trust the in-laws? Better not answer that!

The pain in his right knee was dulling a little now. Must have been standing up too much today. What would it be like in ten years time? Not like the image he used to have of nice old people, with their white hair and sticks. He hadn't realised how tiring it could be – having pain all the time.

He knew that Mr Choleric had arthritis in most of his joints, as well as his poorly controlled blood pressure, and his prostatic enlargement. Apart from the physical deterioration, there was real feeling of a person who had lost his former status, who had changed from being a person of some consequence to someone of no account, at least in his own eyes. Was this what retirement held in store? 'It's no fun getting old, is it, doctor?' was a phrase used frequently by some of the patients, but never by Mr Choleric. Was it pride that stopped him from saying it?

He always felt at a loss to answer this question which, he felt, was not entirely rhetorical. Was it true that there was nothing positive to which one could look forward? How could he reassure people who were further on in their journey through life than he was himself? How could *he* relate to such a depressing message from the future?

'Don't tell me – he's a Celt!' says Donald.
'How do you know?'
'Glass always half empty,' says Donald. 'preferably one in each hand!'
'Very funny,' says Liam, 'but I prefer to think that I come from a line of people steeped in artistic tradition.'
'You should all get a life,' says Donald. 'Go and watch a good game of football!'

Dr Susan was up late with her revalidation folder. She needed three things to work on for the learning plan. All she could think of was how to cope with the 'heartsink' patients like Mrs Liszt. But no, that was out of date. There weren't supposed to be patients like that any more, just 'heartsink' doctors. That meant it was all her fault, and tomorrow she was having an annual appraisal with Dr Avenger, the Clinical Governance lead. They said he was very serious and asked for evidence for everything. They also said that there was no 'pass' or 'fail', but she wasn't convinced. Somewhere in the recesses of the Primary Care Trust, there was sure to be a dossier on everybody, and she wanted to get a good grade. Sometimes she wondered where this drive to be the best came from. Was it mainly from within herself or was she still trying to please her parents? Now, of course, she was keen for her own children to get good grades. That was why she helped with their homework, and worked longer hours to help pay for their school fees. And so the cycle went on? She glanced quickly at her husband who was still asleep in front of the television.

How to address the learning need? She had recently seen something about a Balint group starting up. Maybe this was a way to begin to understand patients who were frequent attenders. She remembered reading something about it for the MRCGP. You had to give them a long interview, she thought. Already things were very tight at the surgery. Long interviews were probably impractical, but there was also a quicker method, she seemed to remember – the 'flash' or something like it. Like a sudden deep understanding, they had said. Connected with Freud, too, wasn't it? She wasn't at all sure she liked the sound of that, but maybe if it helped her with Mrs Liszt? The main problem was going to be finding time for regular meetings, probably in the evening and in the city, fifteen miles away.

'What an amazing professional attitude,' says Liam.
'Scares me to death!' says Donald.
'What does?'
'The sheer efficiency for one thing,' says Donald. 'but I am worried about these doctors getting the right balance in their lives.'
'You mean between professional work, family and leisure?' says Liam. 'I'm sure that's an area to be covered in her appraisal by Dr Avenger.'
'Well, I hope he's properly trained, this Avenger fellow,' says Donald. 'It seems to me that he's taking on quite a problem. What about all the drinking and depression? How long do they get for this appraisal thing?'
'About a couple of hours.'
'Wow!' says Donald.

'Any other business?' said Dr Strait, gathering up the agenda and his papers.
They were all very busy but, as usual, felt a reluctance to leave the meeting and re-engage with the paperwork and visits.
'You're looking a bit tired, Sue,' said Dr Shorts, observing the lack of a ready smile on her features.
'I'm permanently tired,' said Dr Susan, 'but I guess it's normal isn't it?'
'Don't know how you do it all,' said Dr Shorts. 'Have you got any holiday coming up?'

'Not soon enough!' said Dr Susan. 'But holidays aren't exactly a rest either.'

'I thought you had it all,' said Dr Strait; 'a career, children . . . and all the patients love you.'

'Oh come off it Dai! Don't you remember when your children were young? I suppose your wife did everything, didn't she?'

'I'm sorry to say she did, but I was on call a lot of nights and weekends. Didn't see much of the kids when they were growing up, and I've always regretted it.'

'That's sad,' said Dr Susan. 'It's good that there's less time taken up with out of hours these days, but I seem to be working extra hard for the children when I do arrive home. My husband doesn't get much of a look in – and as for me . . .'

Dr Strait fingered the catch on his briefcase. There was a silence, broken at length by Dr Shorts:

'Reminds me of a trainers' course I went on once. We had to draw pie charts –

you know the sort of thing; circles divided up into segments that represent your life. I remember that I had two huge segments for work and family, and a very tiny slice for what they called "me-time". Felt like it was being squashed between the other two.'

'Just how I feel,' said Dr Susan. 'Nothing else but a workhorse!'

'Funnily enough,' said Dr Shorts, 'everyone else had made a similar chart – and they seemed to think it was all right, that being a professional made it all right somehow. But I didn't think it was, and I still don't.'

'Perhaps I'm being selfish?' said Dr Susan.

'I blame Generation X,' said Dr Strait.

'The "me-time" is very important though,' said Dr Shorts. 'It's your own self that you put into any other situation, whether it's your job or your marriage, or anything else. If you don't look after it, like watering a plant, it starts to wither; then you're not much use to anybody, patients included.'

'All very well, Simon,' said Dr Strait, 'but there's work to be done. It might be worth organising an evening meeting around this topic though.'

'Just help me to understand,' says Donald, 'why these doctors are all so oppressed.'

'Partly it's the age time-bomb,' says Liam.

'The age what?'

'More and more old people,' says Liam, 'with more and more medical and social problems.'

'And not enough doctors?'

'Not enough to deliver what is being asked of them, at any rate,' says Liam.

'What is being asked, then?'

'Well, the other part of the problem is that expectations keep going up. It seems as though society is driven by technology and material wants.'

'Everyone wants to live for ever!' says Donald.

'In perfect health!' says Liam.

'And pay no tax!' says Donald.

'Could it be heaven they're wanting?' says Liam. 'Anyway you saw a sample of it in those case histories.'

Eventually Simon, Susan and Dai had their evening meeting, with a takeaway, and soft drinks because they were all driving back. Susan talked about her ideas for joining a Balint group, but Dai was not impressed.

'You mean you want to delve even more into their psychological problems?' said
  Dr Strait, affecting surprise. 'You're already the most popular doctor in the
  practice. What are you trying to achieve?'
'It's because I'm the only female doctor you have,' replied Dr Susan, 'and the
  majority of appointments are for women.'
'Won't be a problem soon,' said Dr Strait. 'I'll retire and you can replace me with a
  woman.'
'Two women, more like,' said Dr Shorts, 'or even two men. Not so many doctors
  want to work full-time.'
'Perhaps they all want to get a life!' said Dr Strait.
'I would go part-time,' said Dr Susan, 'if I didn't need the money. But the reason
  I'm interested in a Balint group is not to uncover more psychological and social
  stuff. People bring it to you anyway. It's impossible to avoid it. I'm sure you
  have the same, but you like to give out this macho impression, in case anyone
  accuses you of being cardigan wearers!'
'With beards and sandals?' interjected Dr Strait, looking at Simon.
'If you want the full stereotype,' replied Dr Susan. 'What does it mean exactly?
  Everyone knows that doctors deal with people as well as with diseases. Some
  prefer one, rather than the other, but we all have to deal with both.'
'I haven't shaved for over 20 years,' said Dr Shorts, 'and I don't intend to start
  now. Everyone had a beard at one time.'
'Including the women!' said Dr Strait.

'I'm thinking Van Dyck portraits,' says Donald.
'Shhhh!' says Liam.

'Just when I thought we were starting to get somewhere,' said Dr Susan, 'you go
  back to being silly again!'
'Okay, okay!' said Dr Shorts. 'As a matter of fact, I have been thinking around this
  area . . .'
'With the trainers' group, no doubt?' enquired Dr Strait, innocently.
'Yes, with the trainers' group, but not the psychoanalytical approach, not Balint
  at any rate,' said Dr Shorts. 'What we were looking at was the combination of
  medicine with study of the Arts.'
'How can you justify that?' asked Dr Strait.
'Well, the trainers are all experienced educators, and they're convinced.'
'Not good enough!' said Dr Susan.
'It's face validity though,' replied Dr Shorts. 'But let me explain.'
'We're listening,' said Dr Strait.
'I'm sure you'll agree that the practice of medicine is science with art,' said
  Dr Shorts.

'Cum scientia caritas,' intoned Dr Strait.

'Quite so,' said Dr Shorts. 'Doctors have to deal with people in a social context . . .'

'What I've just been saying,' agreed Dr Susan.

'Yes, but also doctors are people in their own social context.'

'And?'

'And developing empathy with other people requires the development of self-awareness. It means you have to offer yourself to the patient as another person as well as a doctor.'

'That feels like what I'm doing,' said Dr Susan.

'But there are costs,' said Dr Shorts. 'Each encounter drains you, and leaves less for the next patient, even for your own family.'

'So you need replenishment?'

'Yes, that's very important, but you also need to maintain balance. What I mean is how much science and problem solving against the humanity side of things. You have to switch between different modes of operating according to the needs of the patient.'

'And your own needs, too,' said Dr Strait.

'Well, you have to look after yourself, but not at the expense of the patient.'

'Meaning what exactly?'

'It's the other side of the coin. Instead of being drained, it's possible to feed off the emotions of the patient – especially if you're interested in psychology.'

'I hadn't realised consulting was so dangerous!' said Dr Strait.

'You're being disingenuous, Dai,' said Dr Shorts. It's a complex balance, and I'm sure you are very good at it.'

Dai and Susan exchanged shrugs.

'The key to it is self-awareness and respect for the patient – the two go together.'

'Where do the Arts come in?' asked Dr Susan.

'The Arts reflect human life. They offer us replenishment sometimes, and always the opportunity to grow through development of self-awareness, because of our responses to works of art.'

'By gum!' exclaimed Dr Strait. 'I think I need a proper drink.'

'And also,' continued Dr Shorts, 'the opportunity to engage with psychological and social concerns in a safe environment.'

'Did you read that in a book?'

'Yes,' said Dr Shorts. 'Good, isn't it?'

Before they went home, Simon explained his idea of resurrecting the local GPs' support group, to provide a programme of meetings, some of them on clinical topics. He suggested that part of the time could be spent on 'Arts and Medicine'. Since one of his acquaintances was a practising artist who was also a teacher, a gentle introduction to paintings in the medical context seemed a logical first step.

'Very neat, but will it work?' says Donald.

'It's not so outlandish,' says Liam. ' "Arts and Medicine" has been around for some time, especially in the undergraduate curriculum. Primary care seems to be the last place for it to catch on, rather surprisingly.'

'Sounds like self indulgence for those who are into art anyway,' says Donald. 'Where's the evidence that it helps?'

'Are you talking about randomised controlled trials?' says Liam. 'It's almost impossible to get that sort of evidence for localised clinical interventions. In education it's even more difficult, because there are too many potentially interfering factors, and less chance of meaningful control groups.'

'I rest my case,' says Donald.

'At least try to keep an open mind!' says Liam.

References

1   Middleton J (2000) *The Team Guide to Communication*. Radcliffe Medical Press, Oxford.

CHAPTER 3

The Arts and Medicine movement

People need recognition, not just clinical management. Empathy is elusive and risky. Self-awareness helps the doctor to cope and to be effective. The Arts are a valuable resource in gaining knowledge of self and others.

I think it's time to leave Dr Shorts and his colleagues to organise themselves and their friendly art tutor. Also Donald needs time off to take Liam to that football match. In the meantime, without attempting to be exhaustive or overly academic, I want to try and set the 'Arts and Medicine' scene in context.

My own work with an experienced trainers' group in Leicester, led by Mike Drucquer, began in 2002 with a study of narrative aspects of literature and painting. We were helped by the input of one of the curators at the National Gallery, who explained what was going on in the pictures. Emboldened by our initial success and full of enthusiasm, we expanded our range of activities to include plays, ballet, a musical and an opera (but not football). Also, having sampled the Arts in our own capital, we ventured abroad – to Prague in 2005, and Madrid in 2006. As our extravagance (self-financed, honest!) increased, so did our need to justify this kind of activity to ourselves, and to our partners who had not been invited. Though we were aware that this might not be an entirely new furrow, we wanted to make more of a connection between the works of art and the patients we were seeing on Monday mornings. In short, we were motivated to produce a curriculum with learning points.[1]

However, Undergraduate Departments have been involved in medical humanities since the 1970s. For example, one of my friends, Paul Lazerus (Dept of General Practice and Primary Care) has been working with Felicity Rosslyn (Dept of English) to deliver a module entitled 'The Arts in Medicine' for Leicester-Warwick Medical School, and I have drawn extensively from their paper about this.[2]

The objectives of the module were to enable the student to:

1 'Describe how human experience of a health or sickness issue is contained in and conveyed by one or more forms of the Arts.'
2 'Discuss how this compares to the experiences of yourself and others with patients.'

3 'Reflect on how the above will be of use to you when dealing with patients in your careers and how it has affected your personal and professional development.'

Initially the emphasis was on the written word, to provide a basis for study, with other art forms introduced during the module. Literature is a rich source of accessible material about health, illness, doctors and medical ethics. These can be amplified and brought to life by the subjective insights of authors. For example, Mark Haddon's novel *The Curious Incident of the Dog in the Night-time* was used to stimulate awareness of and issues related to people with autism and Asperger's syndrome.[3]

In their literature review, Lazerus and Rosslyn have indicated that the problems presented by patients go beyond diagnosis and treatment to involve 'other, often more awkward variables – patients' beliefs, concerns and expectations, their social and environmental circumstances, and indeed the very way in which they present their problems.' It is, therefore, necessary for doctors to 'develop their powers of understanding patients in these contexts' and also to develop their own self-awareness. Arts can help this by 'stimulating insight into common patterns of response', by 'highlighting individual differences' and by 'enriching the language and thought of the practitioner.'

Students were asked to choose one area of human illness experience, in a particular arts setting, for in-depth study, and to submit a 3000 word essay for the purpose of assessment. They were also expected to keep a reflective learning journal. Students were supported by seminars, such as the ones listed in 2002:

- introduction and orientation
- poems and learning journals
- introduction to literature and medicine
- information retrieval skills
- images of the doctor in literature
- visit to Museum of Modern Art, Oxford
- death and dying in literature
- images of the artist
- drama workshop
- depression in literature
- music and the mind
- disability in film
- review, reflections and feedback.

Amongst the projects chosen for in-depth study were the following which are relevant to our topic of painting and medicine:

- art therapy – patients' experience of illness expressed by their art
- art and arthritis
- William Blake – his visions, why he had them, and their effect on his work
- life, individuality and death, as perceived by Damien Hirst.

Qualitative evaluation of the module indicated the students' perception that their professional development had been enhanced by studying the Arts and that they would continue to use the Arts to this end. One student bemoaned the emphasis on suffering and felt that 'more happy topics' were needed. This induced the authors to draw a parallel between the lives of artists and the professional experiences of doctors. Written assessments showed that the objectives of the module were achievable by the great majority of students.

According to Lazerus and Rosslyn, 'the module's aim and objectives were geared to producing doctors with an enhanced capacity for understanding the reactions and behaviours of patients, not only to health and sickness, but also toward the doctor to whom they turn for help. Beyond this, it was intended that students would become aware of their own responses and attitudes, and usefully increase their powers of expressing (or when appropriate, suppressing) these.' It also provided the 'opportunity for medical students to be taught by teachers from disciplines outside medicine . . . with obvious benefit in reducing the insularity of medical schools.'

Interesting points from the discussion were:

- 'the cost to the doctor of exposure to others' long-term depression' and the notion that depression lies in wait for most clinicians at some stage of their career
- 'the difficulty of getting access to the patient's inner world'
- 'the medical attitude to death, the tendency to view it as a failure rather than an inevitable factor for us all'
- 'the role assumed by the doctor in donning the white coat.'

Since the module was optional, it is quite likely that students who took part already had a leaning in the direction of the Arts. More than half of them already wrote poetry, painted or played music, and 'several of them commented that the course helped them keep in touch with a self that a medical training left no time for, and which felt in danger of being distorted by constant facts and figures.' On the other hand, it is probable that a majority of entrants to medical school have an interest in humanity as well as science, whether or not that interest is suppressed during clinical training.

Although it is true that the 'humanities beacon' had been lit by the undergraduate teachers a good while ago and, despite the holistic philosophy of vocational training for general practice, I recall the incredulity of a group of trainees who were asked to listen to Barber's Adagio for Strings and reflect on their feelings. This was back in 1983 when I was a 'rookie' course organiser. They told me that they had done the 'Man in Society' module at medical school, and were already 'socially aware'. 'Right', I snapped. 'Next week it's the Red Eye, and the only connection with crying is how you'll feel when you sit the multiple choice!' Actually, as you've probably guessed, I didn't say this, nor even think of it till later.

Years later, I became aware of the writings of John Salinsky on 'Medicine and Literature' in *Education for General Practice*, now *Education for Primary Care* –

known as the 'Green Journal'. These have now been collected in two anthologies.[4,5] Salinsky's best school subjects were Biology and English – just like me. Unlike some of us, he continued to read literature during his medical training. I suspect that this was partly a form of escapism from the world of medical facts and figures, but later he found resonance with the lives of patients he met in general practice. This helped in recognising patients as human beings, resembling old friends in books, and in regarding them 'in a more benign, forgiving and tolerant way.' Again, in the author's own words: 'as soon as I recognise characters in the surgery as belonging to the same human family as my friends from the classics, my anger and frustration dissolve, and a nicer part of my personality is able to emerge. If you were to call all this an enhanced capacity for empathy, I should not disagree.'

Salinsky makes a strong case for reading the classics, in preference to lighter or unproven fare: they are better written and reliable (possibly having more reliable insights into people and their lives); their quality is proved by their survival over time and culture.

The first offering is Franz Kafka's *A Country Doctor*, which was adopted as an introduction to 'Medicine and the Arts' by my own trainers' group. This is, obviously, a story about a doctor who shares some of the same uncertainties and dilemmas as present day general practitioners. It is also curiously dreamlike, and appears to have multiple layers of meaning, depending on your interpretation. Information about Kafka's life is supplied, in an attempt to explore his possible motivations and feelings. These insights have considerable relevance to the argument encapsulated in this book.

Salinsky goes on to tackle such heavyweights as Tolstoy's *Anna Karenina*, Emily Bronte's *Wuthering Heights*, Dostoyevsky's *The Brothers Karamazov* and Flaubert's *Madame Bovary* (the latter was also adopted by my trainers' group, because one of the central characters is a doctor). As the author points out though, many of the books are not about doctors as such, but doctors and illnesses tend to creep in. Moreover, the doctors often don't behave very well, which may stimulate discussion around medical ethics.

Some readers may wish to see a more definite connection between lessons from literature and how to manage specific cases. Nevertheless, the author's point, that it has the potential to enhance empathy and respect for patients in a global sense, is well made. How do you prove it? Given the difficulty in demonstrating benefits of clinical interventions, without recourse to randomised controlled trials and large numbers of patients (and doctors), we should perhaps not be too defensive about this. There is still a great deal of medical practice which is based on tradition, rather than firm evidence.

From the early 1970s, Salinsky has been a member of a 'Balint' group, looking at doctor–patient relationships.[6] This group extended the traditional scope of study from these relationships, and the stories of patients, to exploration of the doctors' feelings and defences. The work of the group has been chronicled in collaboration with Paul Sackin.[7]

The authors have attached the text of a lecture, from the Journal of the Balint Society, given by Tom Main in 1978. In it he states that:

'the trained, disciplined use of subjectivity as a source of scientific information is rare; in the service of medicine moreover it will inevitably often involve us in pain.'

'. . . how much pain can the GP stand and yet retain his capacity to think?'

'the "flash of mutuality" – clearly offers the least strain, for it only occurs if the doctor is ready and in good shape at the time.'

'. . . if we cease to be censorious about defences in ourselves and our colleagues . . . we can hope to replace non-thinking automatic, rigid procedures of careful encounter and defence by thoughtful, elastic and adaptive, deliberate techniques.'

Salinsky and Sackin go on to talk about warning signs of defences, such as irritability, retreat to procedures and protocols, and preoccupation with time. They stress the importance of self-awareness in combination with listening properly to patients, both in medical education and continuing professional development.

Mead and Bower[8] have proposed a conceptual framework for 'patient-centredness' with five key dimensions:

1 biopsychosocial (known as the triple diagnosis)
2 patient-as-person (patient's experience of illness)
3 sharing power and responsibility
4 the therapeutic alliance (Balint's 'mutual investment company')
5 doctor-as-person.

In their review of the literature, Mead and Bower quote McWhinney's description of the patient-centred approach as one where 'the physician tries to enter the patient's world, to see the illness through the patient's eyes'.

We perhaps nod wisely but, in truth, this is impossible isn't it? 'I know just how you feel' is an expression which might be construed as insulting. My individual experience is unique. How dare you attempt to usurp it! The philosophical consequence of this point of view is what Sartre calls *anguish*[9] – the realisation that the individual is alone, and unable to understand others (or to be understood by them), *except by projecting his own experience* (my italics).

By projecting his own experience and offering himself as a 'universal man', the iconic country doctor, John Sassal, attempted to reach his patients as a person instead of just a technician. This was an about-face, as he had been a surgeon before going into general practice. I have a mischievous thought that Martin Clunes' character ('Doc Martin' on ITV1) might resemble a much earlier stage of the transformation. *A Fortunate Man*: the book about Sassal's life as a GP, by a novelist and a photographer – recently re-issued by the Royal College of General Practitioners[10,11] – has been a major influence on a generation of doctors.[12] However, some of the new generation have had the temerity to question the wisdom of trying to be all things to all people, especially in an age where doctors are tending to relinquish continuity of care in favour of their own personal and family lives,[13,14] It now becomes possible to talk of Sassal's depression and suicide, though we don't know whether his approach to work was a cause or a symptom.

So the message is that subjective insight into patients' experiences is valuable, but it comes at a cost. How does the doctor cope with the strain and the pain, and do the 'housekeeping'[15] to be ready for the next patient? Enter the Arts and Medicine at postgraduate level.

Elaine Powley and Roger Higson[16] have compiled a course organiser's handbook, complete with music CD, for the use of different arts media in medical education. They offer a clear structure with group exercises, to enhance awareness through narrative, poetic language, music and feelings, looking at pictures and objects, and alternative selves through role-play. The authors also assert that participants in their courses 'often departed happy, excited and fulfilled' through discovery of the feelingful part of themselves.

Peter Barritt's book, *Humanity in Healthcare*,[17] also arises from his work as a course organiser, but is very different in character. This is an intensely rich, thoughtful and academic work, which draws on a great variety of sources. Beginning with the philosophy and politics of healthcare, he moves on to a consideration of suffering from a number of different angles, including the spiritual. The final section deals with the concept of healing, and not just for patients: this includes time for the self and family, professional fulfilment, and the value (and risks) of *vulnerability* (my italics) in relation to professional virtue.

The bulk of Mary Butterton's *Music and Meaning*[18] consists of interviews with a great range of people about their lives, their relationships with music, and what makes certain works special for them. This is underpinned by a theoretical framework which draws together threads from the philosophy of music, developmental psychology, psychoanalytic thought, and neuroscience. The author, who is a musician and a psychotherapist, presents sound as a universal preverbal experience. Depending on the type of music and the state of mind of the listener, it can be supportive and restorative (as in the womb), or stimulating reflection on and exploration of the outside world. Whether or not it does one or the other is related to 'how we are wired up' as individuals, as well as the circumstances at the time.

I hope the readers (and the authors) will not mind my selective musings on some of the books that have recently become available. Each of us has their own individual reactions to books, as with works of art. It seems to me that practising healthcare professionals are increasingly able to access resources to help them, not only with understanding the points of view of clients and patients, but also with understanding and looking after themselves. The insights are perhaps scattered over a number of sources, and might benefit from being brought together in a more cohesive whole.

My survey of the literature of 'Arts and Medicine' (of which only a selection is quoted here) also reveals the lack of a book on painting in its own right, resourced by a practising artist. The time must be ripe, as the recent James Mackenzie Lecture, on the subject of patient-centred medicine, was illustrated by reproductions of paintings.[19] Fortunately I know just the person for the job.

'Cheer up!' says Liam
'Doh!' says Donald
'But it was a beautiful goal,' says Liam

'Scored by the other side', groans Donald
'Remember – beauty is in the eye of the beholder!' says Liam

References

1 Middleton J and Drucquer M (2006) Arts and medicine in postgraduate medical education. *Education for Primary Care*. (In press).

2 Lazerus PA and Rosslyn FM (2003) The Arts in Medicine – setting up and evaluating a new special study module for students at the Leicester-Warwick Medical School. *Medical Education*. **37**(6): 553–59.

3 Haddon M (2004) *The Curious Incident of the Dog in the Night-time*. Vintage Books, New York.

4 Salinsky J (2002) *Medicine and Literature: the doctor's companion to the classics*. Radcliffe Medical Press, Oxford.

5 Salinsky J (2004) *Medicine and Literature, Volume 2, the doctor's companion to the classics*. Radcliffe Medical Press, Oxford.

6 Balint M (1964) *The Doctor, his Patient and the Illness* (2e). Pitman, London.

7 Salinsky J and Sackin P (2000) *What Are You Feeling, Doctor? Identifying and avoiding defensive patterns in the consultation*. Radcliffe Medical Press, Oxford.

8 Mead N and Bower P (2000) Patient-centredness: a conceptual framework and review of the empirical literature. *Social Science and Medicine*. **51**: 1087–110.

9 Sartre J-P (1957) *Being and Nothingness* (trans. Barnes HE). Methuen, London.

10 Berger J and Mohr J (1967) *A Fortunate Man: the story of a country doctor*. Penguin, London.

11 Berger J (2005) *A Fortunate Man: the story of a country doctor*. RCGP, London.

12 Feder G (2005) A Fortunate Man: still the most important book about general practice ever written. *Br J Gen Pract*. **55**: 246–7.

13 Hutt P (2005) GPs – fortunate or unfortunate? *BMJ Careers*. **September**: 121.

14 Cuthbert CR (2005) An unfortunate man (Letter). *Br J Gen Pract*. **55**: 715.

15 Neighbour R (2004) *The Inner Consultation: how to develop an effective and intuitive consulting style* (2e). Radcliffe Publishing, Oxford.

16 Powley E and Higson R (2005) *The Arts in Medical Education: a practical guide*. Radcliffe Publishing, Oxford.

17 Barritt P (2005) *Humanity in Healthcare: the heart and soul of medicine*. Radcliffe Publishing, Oxford.

18 Butterton M (2004) *Music and Meaning: opening minds in the caring and healing professions*. Radcliffe Medical Press, Oxford.

19 Stewart M (2005) Reflections on the doctor-patient relationship: from evidence and experience. *Br J Gen Pract*. **55**: 793–801.

CHAPTER 4

Stories about people

Patient-centred practice includes attempting to understand the whole person and their illness experience. One way is to listen to the patient's own account (or to consider the 'story' which may be contained in a painting). Another is to start from the case notes (or the painting) and to try to tell the story from the other person's viewpoint.

Refreshments were being cleared away and the hubbub of 'shop talk' was beginning to subside. Dr Shorts stood up and cleared his throat.

'I hope you've brought the October BJGP with you,' he said. 'If not, I have a few spare photocopies of the paper by Moira Stewart, though the pictures will only be in monochrome'.[1]

'What's all this?' says Donald.
'It was mentioned at the end of the last chapter,' says Liam, 'whilst we were watching your team lose.'
'Don't remind me!' says Donald.
'Anyway, she's a Canadian professor who gave the annual James Mackenzie lecture. It was all about patient-centred clinical method.'
'Riveting, I'm sure,' says Donald.
'Yes it is!' says Liam. 'Now pay attention!'

'On page 794, you will see a box with the six components of the patient-centred method. I think the first two are particularly relevant to the subject for this evening':

* Exploring both disease and the patients' illness experience
* Understanding the whole person

'We have already done some work on narrative in literature, and how that compares with the stories that patients tell us.'
'If we let them!' Dr Strait interjected.

Dr Shorts looked slightly ruffled: 'In case nobody has noticed, my senior partner is honouring us with his presence.'

'Excuse me,' said Dr Susan. 'I couldn't make that meeting, unfortunately. Is it possible to fill me in a bit?'

'As far as I understand it, narratives are subjective accounts – stories by people taking part in the action, or by the novelist, writing in character. They are often quite different from the contents of a patient's medical record, or a history book, both of which are trying to present an objective view. You could have a look at John Launer's book on narrative[2] – there's a copy in the practice library. I've also brought along Powley and Higson's practical guide,[3] which has a useful chapter called 'It's my story'. At the end of the chapter you'll find an exercise using patients' notes, where you are invited to write the story from the point of view of the patient. I certainly found that one an eye-opener!'

'Thank you, Simon,' said Dr Susan.

'Now, going back to the same page of Stewart's paper: Figure 2 shows a painting by Robert Pope, called *Visitors*. Although the reproduction is small, I think you'll agree that the image is striking.' The doctors were nodding their heads, looking at the picture of visitors around a patient's bed.

'The perspective is weird,' said Dr Susan, 'though I suppose it's logical, given that the picture is from the patient's viewpoint.'

'It's like looking through the lens of a camera, rather than the way you might see it in reality,' said Dr Strait. 'Still, it reminds me of the way everything seemed distorted when I had a high fever as a kid. Measles, I think it was.'

'The patient would have a story to tell though – don't you agree?' said Dr Shorts. 'You could tell your story, Dai, as a child with measles.'

'How long have you got?' said Dr Strait.

'Not only that,' said Dr Susan, 'but I want to hear the story of the woman visitor on the patient's left, who's holding out the book.'

'You could perhaps tell it for her,' said Dr Shorts.

'But that would be speculation!'

'It's all we have to go on – speculation based on our own experience. Unless you think that the artist's own account, on the opposite page, is helpful.'

'Pretty opaque, I would say,' said Dr Strait.

'You could look at the other pictures,' said Dr Shorts, 'especially Figure 1, *Sparrow*, on page 794, where the man lying on the bed is watching the bird singing, through the window.'

'Or Figure 5 on page 796, *Mr S is told he will die*,' said Dr Strait.

'They're all like snapshots,' said Dr Susan. 'It's as though we've arrived in the middle of their stories.'

'Don't you think that's like case-notes, sometimes,' said Dr Shorts. 'Where have they come from to here?'

'And where are they going?' said Dr Susan.

'Well these reproductions are too small and cartoon-like,' said Dr Shorts, 'but our art tutor resource has been setting up the projector whilst we have been talking, and so without further ado . . .'

The following three paintings are in the National Gallery, London.

www.nationalgallery.org.uk

Go to: Collections – Full Collection Index – Select first letter of artist's surname – click on 'image', and again to enlarge it. Or look in the list of references.[4]

The first image shows *The Execution of Lady Jane Grey*, by Paul Delaroche (1833). Lady Jane Grey was the great-granddaughter of Henry VII. Following the death of Edward VI in 1553 she reigned as queen for nine days before being disposed of by the Catholic supporters of Mary Tudor, tried for treason and beheaded at Tower Hill in 1554. I quote from *A Companion to Charnwood Forest*:[5] 'The amiable victim of others' ambition. She was in the bloom of her youth, graceful and pretty … most amiable and unaffected, quiet, modest, and attached to her young husband and to domestic duty.' (According to Roger Ascham in *The Scholemaster*, treated strictly and with physical cruelty by her parents, she took refuge in books and learning.)

'Wyatt's ill-managed insurrection induced Mary to believe that the life of Lady Jane was incompatible with her own safety; and in February 1554, a week after Wyatt's overthrow, Mary signed her death warrant, and that of her husband, Lord Guilford Dudley.'
Jane waved her husband farewell from the window of the Tower.
'Her Christian fortitude enabled her to bear calmly the agony of seeing her husband's headless body carried past, and to approach the block prepared for her own death.'
She is reported to have made the following speech: 'Good people, I come hither to die, and by law I am condemned to the same. The fact, indeed, against the queen's highness, was unlawful, and the consenting thereto by me, but touching the procurement and design thereof by me, or on my behalf, I do wash my hands in innocency before God and the face of you good Christian people this day.'
I see you're all stunned into silence.
The group continued to be silent for about half a minute.
'That picture is just so dramatic!' said Dr Shorts. 'I can hardly bear to look at it!'
'Melodramatic, I call it,' said Dr Strait.
'It certainly has impact, even without hearing any of the story,' said Dr Susan, 'but what strikes me is how she's been a victim all her life.'

The blindfolded Lady Jane, centre stage, is being guided to the block. On her right, in the background, one lady-in-waiting offers up prayers, the other turns away in denial. On her left stands the executioner, with his face visible, leaning on his axe. The observer is very close to, and on the same level as the action.

'That man with the axe,' said Dr Shorts. 'He looks like somebody's father – I don't believe he can actually do it!'

'It makes me think of victims of atrocities in present times,' said Dr Strait, 'and how some of them are examined by doctors to make sure they are fit for the procedure.'

'I see,' said Dr Susan. 'Like being an agent of the state?'

'As we all are,' said Dr Strait, darkly.

Well, I'm not sure where this discussion is leading but, since you seem to be interested in the executioner, you might like to consider writing the narrative from his point of view. Also, guys, I'm afraid he *did* do it.

'They've all gone soft in the head!' says Donald.

'Why do you say that?' says Liam.

'It's nineteenth century eroticism, pure and simple!' says Donald. 'Bondage in fact, with that blindfold! You can see how that Shorts fellow likes them – young, helpless and long red hair!'

'Perhaps you should cool down as well,' says Liam, 'and wait for the chapter on paint language.' (*See* Chapter 7.)

For the second image, we go back two centuries to *Belshazzar's Feast*, Rembrandt van Rijn 1636–8:

The subject comes from chapter five of the Old Testament Book of Daniel. At a feast the idolatrous King of Babylon uses precious utensils looted from the Temple of God at Jerusalem. Suddenly the hand of God appears, writing the fatal words in Hebrew, which translated mean: 'You have been weighed in the balance and found to be wanting', referring to Belshazzar's judgement by God and imminent death. At this the Old Testament tells us 'the king's countenance was changed . . . and his knees smote one against the other'. He rises in terror, his gold chain swinging, as he knocks over the goblet behind him.[4] Above the king's outstretched left arm, illuminated in a circle of light, a disembodied hand is writing the dread words. Below his arm, a bare-shouldered female figure grasps the neck of the goblet as it falls, the contents flowing downwards. On his right, in the lower quarter of the picture, three seated figures start back in surprise.

Have you ever been caught doing something you shouldn't have?

'First tell me if this is on camera,' said Dr Strait. 'But seriously, it makes me think of all those people binge-drinking and taking drugs.'

'And we are the ones writing on the wall, perhaps,' said Dr Shorts.

'But they're not listening, are they?' said Dr Susan, 'And I don't put myself in the position of God!'

'I'm not sure there is one, anyway,' said Dr Strait. 'There's too much suffering in the world.'

Before you all get carried away with this subject, can I gently point out another opportunity – to write the story from the king's point of view or, if you prefer, from that of a patient you know, who has been confronted with a lifestyle which might have fatal consequences.

'That's a shame,' says Donald. 'I was just settling back to enjoy it: religion and politics – always good for a bit of fisticuffs!'

Ahem! Well, the third image is *Samson and Delilah*, Peter Paul Rubens c.1609.

This painting was commissioned to hang in the 'Great Saloon' of Nicolaas Rockox who was the burgomaster of Antwerp.

The story: Delilah was offered 1100 pieces of silver by the Philistines to discover the secret of Samson's superhuman strength, which would lead to their capture of him. She seduces him, which results in his confiding to her that his strength lies in his hair – if it's cut off he will lose his strength. Delilah betrays him and the barber cuts off Samson's hair as he sleeps, exhausted by sex. Through the door, we see the Philistines in the distance, waiting to capture Samson.

'Wow!' says Donald. 'Look at those boobs! Perhaps I should visit the National Gallery more often!'
'And look at Samson's muscles,' says Liam.
'Speak for yourself!' says Donald.

'Whose story should we write here?' said Dr Susan. 'I don't think the earth exactly moved for Delilah, do you?'
'Maybe he needs a prescription?' said Dr Strait. 'How old do you think he is?'
'About 20 years younger than you!' said Dr Susan.
'Now, now – children!' said Dr Shorts. 'But there's a whole raft of associations for doctors, apart from erectile dysfunction: psychosexual problems, infidelity . . .'

Well guys, we've had plenty of reaction to the possible stories evoked by these paintings. Just wait till we get onto the paint language, but not this evening. Before we close – here's something more personal – *Tree of Life I* (2003, Plate 2) (exhibited in the Lorenzo Lotto School of Art in conjunction with the Venice Biennale 2005):

This painting charts the first 23 years of my married life. It was inspired by the Venetian artist, Lorenzo Lotto's *Virgin and Child with Saints* (1539, Cingoli, Pinacoteca Civia Italy).

For image – Google: Lorenzo Lotto virgin saints 1539 Cingoli.
Or : www.artrenewal.org/asp/database).

Lotto's painting has 15 narrative roundels which depict the 15 standard scenes from the lives of Christ and the Virgin. Below these are a number of saints surrounding the Virgin and Child, each holding a characteristic attribute or gesticulating.

I liked the power of the symmetry and wanted to continue the discourse in a personalised contemporary setting. I took the 15 roundels (*see* Plate 4), used them to depict scenes from our family life, and set them against a different tree backdrop, three trees in my case, to represent the Trinity.

'So, is this some kind of religious statement?' said Dr Strait.
'I don't think it has to be, necessarily,' said Dr Susan. 'Many people, who aren't religious, appreciate Bach's settings of the Passion. Other composers have followed that tradition of setting religious texts, whatever their personal beliefs. This painting might just be following in the footsteps of Lorenzo Lotto.'

I shall now explain the imagery in further detail but, before doing so, would just like to point out that there are weaknesses in this painting. The scale of the roundels, being only 2″ across, is too small for accurate detail on the group scenes. The figures at the bottom are rather 'wooden'. There is virtually no expressive paint language; the meaning is derived cognitively, through imagery alone. Addressing these problems gave rise to the much larger *Tree of Life II* (*see* Plate 8) a year later, but far from solving everything, new problems arose. That's the nature of being a painter though – it's a parallel journey, with its own ups and downs, discoveries, joys and disappointments – in our quest to understand. Truth and beauty go hand in hand.

'Ah, but what is truth?' says Donald.
'You've said that before,' says Liam.
'But not in this book!' says Donald.

'To be honest, I thought that the figures were painted that way to mimic a more primitive style,' said Dr Susan.
'Artists are their own worst critics, aren't they?' said Dr Shorts.

The tree imagery is an old one, going back to medieval times – branches representing facets of ideas, relationships, or continuity. In contrast to family trees where the connections are clear and logical, the arrangement here is more ambiguous, less specified, allowing for some individual response in the observer. Nevertheless, the central three (symbolic in itself) roundels represent central tenets: the marriage; God (represented through our daughter's first holy communion); the home (we live at number three, and the front door imagery also forms a cross). These tower directly above my head.

Top row, left of centre: our first-born child, born dead. They wrapped her up in a white gown and handed me this photograph.

Top row, far left: the christening of the first live baby (a boy), wearing the gown worn by me and my brothers, and all the previous generation – fellow travellers through life and time.

Top row, right of centre: me, just over a year later, peering into our daughter's incubator, the day after delivery. Our children spent a total of 20 weeks in SCBU between them.

Top row, far right: daughter and son sheltering from hot sun at Youlgreave, Derbyshire, where we often went walking.

Middle row, far left: Burnham Overy Staithe, Norfolk, where we took family holidays for 15 years on the trot. Far right: in our rowing boats on the River Soar, at the bottom of our garden.

Middle row, left of centre, our son practising his violin on the patio. Although it was summer, he put on wellies rather than go to the effort of sandals and buckles. Middle row, right of centre: Easter Day – everyone's chocolate eggs are lined up on the patio table.

Bottom row, far left: Christmas Dinner. Left of centre: our daughter and son, all dressed up at one of my brothers' second wedding on HMS Warrior at Portsmouth. Right of centre: Anthony doing a magic trick – he has since become a semi-professional magician, earning his way through university. Far right – four of the cousins together on Southsea beach.

'Just as I told you!' said Dr Strait. 'She's a believer.'

'What if she is?' said Dr Susan. 'So was Bach, by all accounts.'

'I don't like to be preached at,' said Dr Strait.

'Doesn't sound like preaching so far,' said Dr Shorts. 'Anyway, Dai, we have to respect our patients' views, no matter how different they are from our own.'

'Therefore, we must try and understand them, too,' said Dr Susan. 'Let's make an effort to understand this painting. I think it helps to know about the story behind it.'

And now to the figures below (*see* Plate 3). Far left, my husband and the co-author of this book, in hiking gear. Next to him, Rachael, our daughter (she should have been holding some animal attribute, as she is now a vet student). Then, Anthony – never one to enter a room quietly. Here he is, doing another trick, whereby many items are taken from a bag which was previously shown to hold nothing. 'O fortuna' refers to the life we are dealt out, as it were. What is the fortune of these two? He wears vermilion, clashing with my alizarin crimson, referring to our all too similar personalities. The Venetian carnival mask both hides and presents a persona. This reminds me of Frida Kahlo's self-portraits – how to present the self (*see* Chapter 5).

Myself as Madonna – the 'Christ Child' becomes the palette, a sort of site of birth (of paintings). I hold three brushes, referring again to the Trinity. I wear deep red, the colour of martyrs. My hair becomes fetishistically long and a deeper gold than in reality. Red is also the complementary (on the colour wheel) of the green surroundings, whilst linking with the reds left and right in the figures. The steadfast gaze was meant to be the pivotal point, around which everything else circulates. Why martyr? Well, only that my main life's energy has been spent on supporting others rather than promoting myself, and bearing the costs physically and career-wise. At the time of writing I've had 14 operations, almost all connected with having children. And do I regret this path? Emphatically *no*. Having got so far, it became my duty to see the thing through. So it's not a self-pitying image of martyrdom, but rather a 'well, I'm still here, through thick and thin'. I am not a well-known artist; I am only very low on the academic hierarchy, but I've got a very close, loving, stable family. To me this is progress.

To the right of me: a close friend, our mutual spiritual guide: charismatic, teaching us by example without even realising he was doing so. He died early, influencing us increasingly deeply during the drawn-out illness.

Far right – another close friend, equally charismatic, but in a zany way. She taught me painting in my first degree, and has subsequently become a close friend of the family, and one of my very few soulmates. Reaching much further than teaching painting as such, she somehow managed to put me in touch with the self I never knew until I met her, flying in the face of all my upbringing. I could tell you many amusing stories, but her underlying teachings were to savour the joyful moment (no matter how dire the general circumstances), to disobey all unnecessary rules automatically and to remain alive to the recognition of visual beauty at all times.

Well, that's the story behind the picture. And now you also know a little about the artist behind it.

'Thank you for that very thought-provoking presentation about painting and narrative,' said Dr Shorts. 'I think we have made some interesting connections between the pictures and issues that might concern our patients, such as child-birth, the family and roles, death, bereavement and spiritual belief. It also seems to me that we have started to move onto the next topic, which is stories about the artists themselves, their feelings and motivations.'

'Yes,' said Dr Susan. 'It's relatively simple when pictures tell a story, but what about portraits or even abstract works?'

'Coming soon, on a PowerPoint presentation near you,' said Dr Strait.

'I can see that doctors can make all sorts of connections with patients and medical prac-tice, from stories suggested by paintings,' says Donald, 'but they could do that by reading stories, or just by thinking about their patients as people.'

'That's true,' says Liam, 'but the idea is to increase their sensitivity to the ideas and experience of other people.'

'But why paintings?' says Donald. 'Comic strips might do just as well.'

'Difficult to do Rothko as comic strip!' says Liam. 'Anyway, you'll meet him in the next chapter.'

'Oh no!' says Donald.

The transition from painting as illustration to paint as communication in itself, is explored partly through the painting *Tree of Life II* (*see* Plate 8), in Chapter 7.

References

1   Stewart M (2005) Reflections on the doctor-patient relationship: from evidence and experi-ence. *Br J Gen Pract*. **55**: 793–801.

2   Launer J (2002) *Narrative-based Primary Care: a practical guide*. Radcliffe Medical Press, Oxford.

3   Powley E and Higson R (2005) *The Arts in Medical Education: a practical guide*. Radcliffe Publishing Ltd, Oxford.

4   MacGregor N (1997) *Making Masterpieces*. BBC Education Production, London.

5   Anonymous (1858) *A Companion to Charnwood Forest*. Simpkin, Marshall & Co, London.

CHAPTER 5

Stories about painters

When paintings do not apparently contain narratives, another way of inferring mean-ing is to find out about the artists who painted them. To a greater or lesser extent, the life of a painter is art. Whether or not it is overtly autobiographical, every work of art reflects the inner core of the person who produced it. Artists' lives are often colourful, but then so are the lives of some patients. They contend with fundamental issues that we all have to face. In attempting to understand what they are trying to communicate, we can learn more about ourselves through our reactions, and thus enhance our abil-ity to understand others.

In the last meeting, I began to tell you a little about myself and about my family. That was because it was the subject of the painting *Tree of Life I*, or least it was on one level. On another level it goes back to the tradition of Lorenzo Lotto, and pain-ters in that genre, to reflect how this way of looking at life might resonate with us today. At least it attracted attention, at the recent Venetian exhibition, from members of the Lorenzo Lotto Art School. Although two of my works, reproduced here, are what you might call family album pictures, most of my paintings are not overtly self-referencing. This is in marked contrast with the first artist about whom I would like to say a few words.

Frida Kahlo (Mexican: 1910–1954)

For a number of self-portrait paintings, including *The Broken Column*:
Google: enter 'Frida Kahlo self portraits' and click on 'images'.
For *The Broken Column* only:
Google: enter 'Frida Kahlo Broken Column' and click on 'images'.
Accessed 22 January 2006

Frida Kahlo's life and art were determined primarily by an acute awareness of her own body. This awareness began at the age of six when she was stricken with polio. This resulted in a withered leg which she hid all her life with full length clothing, whether Mexican costume or through cross-dressing. At 18 she was involved in a horrendous traffic accident which resulted in multiple fractures of the pelvis and vertebrae. Included in the injuries were a deep abdominal wound caused by a metal rod entering through the hip and exiting through the groin (she is reported to have said that this is how she lost her virginity), multiple fractures of the right foot and dislocation of an elbow. As if this wasn't enough, she also had spina bifida, which caused progressive ulceration of her legs and feet. Throughout her life she suffered relapses, undergoing over 30 different operations and often having to wear constricting casts and metal corsets. *The Broken Column* (1944, Museo Dolores Olmedo Patino, Mexico City) is one of her self-portraits dominated by the physical trauma she had experienced.[1] Her abdominal wounds rendered her unable to bear children – several miscarriages and 'therapeutic abortions' ensued.

'Too much information!' says Donald
'Shhh!' says Liam

Kahlo stated: 'I paint because I need to.'[2]
    There were also other problems. She had a passionate and tempestuous relationship with Diego Rivera, a well-known muralist. They were both unfaithful, Kahlo with both men and women. They married, divorced, then married and divorced again.

'Like the Burtons,' says Donald.
'Who?'
'You know – the film people, Richard and Liz. Always getting divorced and remarried.'
'She had an affair with Trotsky,' says Liam.
'Who did? Liz Taylor?'
'No, Frida Kahlo!' says Liam.

Kahlo painted over 40 self-portraits. When asked why so many, she answered: 'Because I am all alone.'[3]
    Despite major physical problems throughout her life, Kahlo vehemently refused the identity of 'invalid' (what a hero), instead creating an alternative persona: exotic, powerful and proud. Was this denial of reality? Well, why not? What is 'reality' anyway? She set her sights on a more desirable self, and genuinely became it. Kahlo's head, neck and shoulders were her best features, and these she 'flagged' by decorating them. Conversely, all her clothing reached to the ground. So, her life can be seen as a contrasting duality between the exterior persona – constantly reinvented with ornament, costume, and a captivating personality, and the interior artistic persona which fed off her crippled body.
    Germaine Greer,[4] amongst others, has plausibly identified Kahlo as primarily a performance artist, rather than the painter she purported to be. Film footage such as her lying prostrate, lovingly handling a book with heavily ringed fingers, or the powerful direct glance of the charismatic standing Kahlo, can be understood as being exactingly choreographed.

'I have a copy of the August BJGP with the article about Kahlo,'[1] said Dr Shorts.
    'There's a small print of *The Broken Column* in it.'

'Looks like something from a surrealist anatomy textbook!' said Dr Strait. 'I was never keen on women with thick eyebrows – especially if they meet in the middle!'

'She certainly lets it all hang out,' said Dr Susan, 'but I admire her for it.'

Well I'm sure you will agree that, in the case of an artist whose subject is largely the self, it helps to have a little background knowledge of her life, in order to make sense of the paintings. Of course, there were other themes that were important in Kahlo's work, such as the juxtaposition of Mexican folk culture and modern society, but I want to illustrate broad issues and move onto other artists. Next is another woman who is perhaps even more likely to provoke strong reactions.

Tracey Emin (British: 1963–)

For general images including *My Bed*:
Google: enter 'Tracey Emin' and click on 'images'.
For *Scream: a homage to Edvard Munch and all my dead children* stills from the video imagery can be accessed, though this excludes the prolonged scream-ing of which this piece is composed.
Google: enter 'Tracey Emin Scream Edvard Munch Dead Children'.
Edvard Munch's *The Scream*:
Google: enter 'Edvard Munch Scream' and click on 'images'.
Accessed 23 January 2006

Not a painter as such, Emin changes her medium to match her intention, using painting, installation, textiles/appliqué, sculpture, film and neon lights. She is included here because she can be seen as continuing the legacy of Kahlo in post-modern terms.

Emin has welded life and art together in a confessional agenda, covering just about everything, from a bout of herpes to detailing her several abortions. She exposes and humiliates herself, often coming across as a tragic figure, such as in the video performance *Scream: a homage to Edvard Munch and all my dead children*.

Are you sitting comfortably? Then, I'll start the video.

'Please, please, please!' said Dr Susan, rising out of her seat. 'Turn it off – I can't stand it!'

'What's the problem?' said Dr Strait. 'It's only a woman screaming. Not my taste, but it takes all sorts.'

'It's just *horrible*, the thought of what she's screaming about!'

'But is it art?' says Donald.

'At least she gets a reaction,' says Liam.

'I can see where you're trying to lead me,' says Donald. 'It begins with 'Roth' and ends in 'ko'!'

Still, the tormented 'outsider' artist isn't the whole story. Times have changed since Kahlo, and to understand why Emin is so well known (in fact central to the contemporary art world) we need to understand a little about the context within which she flourishes. Patronage has always been inextricably linked with the sort of art being produced. Primary consumership meant Saatchi in her case. The advertising tycoon propelled her to instant fame, along with a number of others by buying many works at increasingly astronomic prices, e.g. *My Bed* for £150,000 in 2000. Secondary consumership means us – buying tickets for talks by Emin, exhibitions, magazines, newspapers, books, journals, watching TV programmes – in which Emin features. Why is she so well known? Because we are voyeuristically supporting her.

'Not me!' says Donald.
'It's always somebody else, isn't it?' says Liam. 'Like people who queue all night for the sales.'
'Never done that either,' says Donald.

Emin left Maidstone College of Art with a First Class degree. She then did a Masters at the Royal College of Art. In 1993 Emin showed 'My Major Retrospective' at White Cube Gallery, Hoxton. In 1997 she contributed to *Sensation*, a major exhibition at the Royal Academy of some of Saatchi's collection. Since then Emin has represented Britain abroad through The British Council, has had exhibitions in this country including Tate Britain, and has been very prominent within the media. What happens in her art from now will be interesting. Can she reinvent herself? The 42-year-old can hardly maintain the 'outsider adolescent' image that got her famous in the first place. What do you make of her, doctors?

'Munchausen's syndrome,' said Dr Strait
'Mmm, I suppose you could see it all as attention-seeking,' said Dr Susan.
'Obviously it's working!' said Dr Strait.
'It's interesting to link these two together as 'performance art', where the script is their own lives,' said Dr Shorts, 'but I think there's more to art than just getting attention, isn't there? I thought artists were driven by something inside.'
'I'm sure they are,' said Dr Susan. 'It's as though they have some kind of fuel burning.'

'Nutters!' says Donald.
'Not all of them!' says Liam.

I have to admit that successful artists tend to be, what shall I say, *alternative*. Normal family life and artistic recognition don't always go together.

'You can say that again!' says Donald.

'Normal family life and being a GP didn't used to go together either!' said Dr Strait.

'It's still not easy for a woman,' said Dr Susan.

'How about the prospect of extended opening hours?' said Dr Shorts. 'Routine consultations, 24/7.'

'Without me!' said Dr Strait. 'I'll retire before it's made illegal!'

Where was I? Artists have difficult lives. Doctors have difficult lives. Both of them are prone to depression, aren't they? Edvard Munch, famous for *The Scream* is a case in point (see previous box).

'That's still a very disturbing picture,' said Dr Susan. 'Even more so in reality, I would imagine.'

'It's easy to forget that,' said Dr Shorts, 'because the image has become little more than a cipher.'

'You mean the new logo for Tony Copperfield's column in *Doctor?*' said Dr Strait.

'Yes, and I've even seen it as a sign outside a pub!' said Dr Shorts.

He said, about his life as an artist: 'Without illness and anxiety I would have been a rudderless ship'.[5] A rudder is used to determine direction, but perhaps he was also referring to the motive force, the fuel that he was burning. Does mental illness fuel art, or does being an artist make you mentally ill? Or is it just a coincidence? Of course, you all know I am coming round to Van Gogh, though controversy still rages over the exact nature of his illness.

Vincent Van Gogh (Dutch: 1853–1890)

www.vangoghmuseum.nl

A post-impressionist painter, Van Gogh was born in northern Brabant, son of a Protestant pastor. In 1869 he began work as an employee of the Goupil Gallery which had been formerly owned by his uncle. In 1873 he was sent to the London branch, as he had been something of an embarrassment in Paris due to lack of diplomacy towards buyers and his own personal views on what art should be. In London he fell in love with the daughter of his landlady – characteristically this was intense and not reciprocated. Influenced by the humanitarian ideas around at the time, Van Gogh abandoned the art business and returned to Holland with the intention of following a religious career. But he didn't fit in with his elders and their religious training either, so left in 1878 and moved to the Borinage, Belgium as a lay-preacher for the miners there. Again, characteristically, he went over the top in his asceticism and self-sacrifice. For example, he gave the very clothes on his back to the miners, and became an embarrassment to the Church who basically sacked him. There followed some months of grave spiritual anguish while he lived like a tramp – a huge embarrassment to most of his family, his father being a respected pastor. But Van Gogh retained his lifelong close relationship with his brother Theo.

From 1881 he decided to become an artist. As usual this was an intense affair right from the start. He often suffered from extreme poverty and undernourishment, but the fact that he coped at all was due to Theo's continual financial support. Over 750 letters from Van Gogh to Theo exist, and these give considerable insight into his artistic aims and mental disturbances. His output as an artist in the remaining nine years of his life was prodigious. He left over 800 paintings and about 850 drawings.

For some months in 1885 he studied painting at the Antwerp Academy, but, characteristically, fell out with the tutors' traditional teaching there and left. From then on he went it alone, painting peasants and workers in a way which expressed their unique dignity – ordinary people had previously tended to be depicted in traditional 'genre' paintings in a rather sentimental way.

In 1886 Van Gogh left Antwerp for Paris – then the epicentre for artistic innovation. His art reflects this stimulating environment, as he experiments with many different ways of painting. It was here that he met Seurat, Pisarro, Degas, Gauguin and Toulouse-Lautrec, amongst others. He became increasingly preoccupied with the expressive use of colour: 'Instead of trying to reproduce exactly what I have before my eyes, I use colour more arbitrarily so as to express myself more forcibly.'[6]

In 1888 Van Gogh settled in Arles where he painted more than 200 canvases in 15 months. During this time he sold no work, was in poverty and suffered recurrent nervous crises with hallucinations and depression. Also, in this period, he cut off a piece of his right ear which he delivered to a prostitute, following a quarrel with Gauguin, who briefly lived with him. Exactly why he did this has been much debated and no definitive answer has resulted.

In 1889 he went at his own request into an asylum near Arles. He continued to paint; much of the work would seem 'disturbed' in terms of normal vision, possibly being indicative of auras in connection with temporal lobe epilepsy. However, this is only one of many speculative diagnoses.

During the last 70 days of his life Van Gogh painted 70 canvases. But his anguish and depression became more acute and on 29 July 1890 he died from a self-inflicted bullet wound.[7] Again, you could read more if you wish – there are numerous sources to choose from – in fact some of us think that his life as the 'tormented artist' of the feature films has become rather a cliché.

'I saw a television programme recently, in which the presenter suggested that Van Gogh's illness had nothing to do with his art, since the paintings were done in between bouts of it,' said Dr Shorts.

'No, I don't believe that,' said Dr Susan, 'because people with bipolar disorder have an altered way of seeing things before they become officially ill. You get hints of it from the way they talk to you, and you think "Oho!", but you can't do anything because they aren't bad enough.'

'Nobody is sure whether he had bipolar disorder or anything else for that matter,' said Dr Shorts.

'Well, suppose he had been put on an SSRI and chlorpromazine, or some other kind of mental handcuffs,' said Dr Strait. 'Do you think he would have painted all those masterpieces?'

'No,' said Dr Shorts. 'and it would have been tragic for him, as well as the rest of us, if he had been stuck with basket weaving.'

'Just look at the intensity of the yellows, and the ferocious way he seems to have made the marks – even on the reproductions,' said Dr Susan.

'I rest my case!' says Donald.

Cliché or not, he obviously still provokes a lot of argument. There is a Van Gogh Museum in Amsterdam – easily accessible on a weekend break, or there are several of his paintings in the National Gallery in London. I suggest you go and spend some time looking at one of them. See what comes out at you, and how much you think his life story or illness has to do with it!

Even if you think post-impressionism, and Van Gogh in particular, is getting rather old hat, maybe the next artist will score more highly on the scale of the bizarre:

Francis Bacon (British: 1909–1992)

Google: enter 'Francis Bacon Three Figures Base Crucifixion' and click on 'images'. You get both the triptych plus details of each panel.

Google: enter 'Francis Bacon Screaming Pope' and click on 'images'. Here there is one of the series in purple predominantly, amongst other associated material.

Born in Dublin, of British parents, Bacon settled to London in 1928. After working as an interior designer Bacon began to paint around 1930 without formal training and with limited success at first. He took part in two group exhibitions at the Mayor Gallery in 1933, had a one-man show at the Transition Gallery in 1934 and took part in the 'Young British Painters' exhibition in the Agnew Gallery in 1937. After that he dropped from sight. In 1944, however, *Three Studies of Figures at the Base of a Crucifixion* exhibited in the Lefevre Galleries (and now in Tate Britain) made him overnight the most controversial painter in post-war Britain. Even so, Bacon did not sell easily until he was in his late forties – his London agent had a vault full of art he could not dispose of. Bacon was swimming against the tide, producing disturbing figurative art at a time when abstract art was popular. Bacon's themes concern violence, suffering, and the aloneness of the human individual.

Outwardly there is little to report about Bacon's life. In his early life it seems that he was abused by grooms at the stables in Ireland – his father bred racehorses near Dublin. Bacon's relationship with his dominant, charismatic father seems to have been traumatic. During the course of his life Bacon had a number of relationships with other men, some of which were exploitative and destructive. Some of the figures in his paintings are portraits of partners, such as George Dyer. Bacon's studio was kept as a chaotic mess. When he did achieve some measure of success, he moved his studio and living quarters to a 'better' area of London, but found this to be an impediment to the production of art. So he moved back again, to the squalor he was used to. The respected late art critic, David Sylvester, made Bacon better understood through a series of searchingly intense interviews during the 1960s, and Bacon's most pertinent commentaries about the nature of art originate from these interviews (*see* Chapter 7).

'These come across as very angry paintings,' said Dr Shorts.
'And he had reasons to be angry, didn't he?' said Dr Susan. 'Like Lady Jane Grey, he's been a victim.'
'I don't have a problem with my own sexuality,' said Dr Strait, 'but I must say this makes me feel a bit uncomfortable. It's lucky all the gays seem to gravitate towards you, Simon.'
'Perhaps it's because they think I'm not so homophobic,' said Dr Shorts.
'I don't think it matters what the artist's sexual orientation was,' said Dr Susan. 'The important issue is that he has been abused, and we've all seen the effect of that on patients.'
'Body image and eating disorders, for example,' said Dr Strait. 'Crucifixion; screaming Popes in cages; pieces of meat hung up – would that be bacon? It looks like he's punishing himself.'

'Do I hear sado-masochism and religion?' says Donald. 'I'm off – at least football is wholesome.'
'Not if some of those chants I heard were anything to go by!' says Liam. 'Anyway, doctors have to deal with all aspects of life, wholesome or not.'

You sure do. I wouldn't swap my job for yours, but now let's look at one of the most famous living painters.

Lucien Freud (British: 1922–)

www.tate.org.uk/britain/exhibitions/freud/work_largeinterior.htm – accessed 29 October 2005)

Freud is of Austrian-Jewish extraction. He came to Britain from Berlin with his parents in 1932, aged 10, and has lived in London ever since. His grandfather was Sigmund Freud.

Outwardly Freud's live seems fairly uneventful. He comes across as deeply introvert in the little media exposure he allows. Both celebrity and recluse, he has an elegant drawing room with Austrian Empire furniture and valuable paintings. Ten metres away is his studio – starkly lit, filthy, cluttered with discarded painting rags and wiped off paint on the walls.

Although a very private man, rumours abound, such as his having multiple children and grandchildren with different partners, and marked gambling habits.

Freud is of world stature, with paintings in many public and private collections globally. His work, which is mainly portraiture, has progressed from the 1940s and 50s, when he used thin wet paint and soft pliant brushes to produce a hard linear realism. Steadily his work has become more brusque, pithier – still the same sort of subjects, but handled in an entirely different way. He is considered to be one of the few modern innovators in the representational tradition. Freud himself stated that he wanted his portraits to be 'of' people, not 'like' them. His paintings often express the human condition of ageing – he underplays facial expression; there is a lack of overt drama or high colour contrast; painterly expression alone rules.[8]

'What does she mean by 'painterly expression'?' says Donald.
'I think it means the way the paint is applied; the language of the paint medium,' says
Liam.
'All Greek to me!' says Donald.

Power relationships with models: power relationships with patients – there's possibly a parallel with Lucien Freud, who's always been powerful (partly because of his grandfather), and doctors who are powerful because of their role in society. Furthermore, his innate personality does come across to me as deeply controlling. There seems to be an unrelenting quest for greater power and inclusion within the Western canon of art. I would argue that everything about his life is subservient to this great need of his: to be recognised by the art world, now and forever – the need to be needed, to be up there with the gods of the art world.

'That's human nature, isn't it?' said Dr Strait. 'It's just like the need that some doctors seem to have to get their names in the BMJ or the BJGP, or to become professors or to be knighted.'
'Not like you then, Dai!' said Dr Shorts.
'You can laugh,' said Dr Strait. 'Just wait till you get the summons from Buckingham Palace!'
'All is vanity in the end,' said Dr Susan. 'What does it all count for?'
'Achievement and recognition, for it gives meaning to life,' said Dr Shorts, 'and it's also a kind of immortality isn't it?'
'What, being a footnote in the BJGP?' said Dr Strait.
'Being in the international canon of Art certainly is,' said Dr Susan.
'But it's interesting how some people maintain that drive for achievement in old age, even to the end of their lives,' said Dr Shorts. 'Lucien Freud is a case in point.'
'Michelangelo, too,' said Dr Susan, 'and Rembrandt.'

'Late self-portraits?' says Donald.
'That's my boy!' says Liam.

'But there are many elderly people around who don't seem to have this kind of energy or drive,' said Dr Strait, 'either because of physical or mental problems, or because they are just out of it. Retired people often don't have the status that once went with their jobs.'

'Like retired doctors?' said Dr Susan

'I'm not sure I want to go there,' said Dr Strait.

'Are you thinking about Mr Choleric?' said Dr Shorts. 'I got the impression from you that he used to be some kind of academic, and now he's just angry and falling to bits.'

'To put it bluntly!' said Dr Strait.

'You're saying his life has no meaning?' said Dr Susan.

'I suppose not,' said Dr Strait.

'But you don't have to be famous or even high status for your life to mean something,' said Dr Susan. 'Just think of all the countless women who have worked for and looked after families. They are great and heroic people in their own way.'

'They are often revered by their extended families,' said Dr Shorts. 'I've seen that, particularly in the Asian community. Also, I think that elderly people tend to be more respected in some eastern cultures.'

'Whereas western culture pursues individuality and eternal youth,' said Dr Strait. 'We're all in denial about death.'

'Reminds me, to some extent, of Mr Tidy,' said Dr Shorts.

'He just wants a doctor's note to put it off indefinitely!' said Dr Strait.

'Not all elderly people are unhappy though,' said Dr Susan. 'I know patients who seem to radiate a feeling of peace and joy, despite the disabilities they have.'

'I agree,' said Dr Shorts. 'How do they manage it? I'd like to find out and put it in a bottle!'

'It must be spiritual,' said Dr Susan. 'One reason why eastern people respect their elders is because they are seen as further along a spiritual journey.'

'You mean that it's their religious faith?' said Dr Shorts.

'Opium!' said Dr Strait. 'Karl Marx said that religion is the opium of the people.'

Guys! I think we're drifting a little from the subject of Lucien Freud.

Consider this: as a general principle, that which is painted equates with that which is written: it comes across as authentic, as one person's enduring truth. But like the writer, the painter is in a position to dominate, marginalise or skew truth. What about others' truths – the unsung heroes, neglected children, discarded models: the forgotten debris in the wake of great masters. Must success cost so much?

'It's quite simple,' says Donald. 'Don't marry an artist!'
'Or a famous footballer?' says Liam.

What Freud (amongst many others in art history) does to the model could be scrutinised in terms of responsibility, at least from a humanitarian perspective. In *Large Interior, Paddington* (1968–9), his young daughter is depicted lying on the floorboards. The accompanying text to the web image states she is having 'an afternoon nap'. Her torso is briefly covered with a vest, the rest naked. Her left hand is obscured as it lies between her naked thighs, and she has a strange unreadable facial expression. The large potted plant that towers over her is dying. Next to that hangs a man's large black jacket. What does it all mean? You can explain it away in terms of an artistic quest for an original composition in terms of dynamism and balance, for example, but something is being done to the vulnerable young child that is outside of her control. The child would presumably have had no say in how she was depicted. I wonder how she feels about this imagery now, as a woman presumably in her late 40s? If she approves, is it partly because her father-painter is famous? Is she under pressure not to put a spanner in the works? Or does she want a part in art history too? Would this make it OK, or is it still an abuse of power?

'Wow!' says Donald. 'Is this art or aversion therapy? Quick, bring me a nice impressionist landscape!'
'Opium, do you mean?' says Liam.

Parallels may be drawn here in terms of power relationships between the artist/model and the doctor/patient in terms of degrees of responsibility. Lucien Freud's role of grand patriarchal figure within his own loose extended family could be seen as roughly equating with the position of the senior GP in relation to his 'family' of junior partners, patients and employees.

'I think I've been missing a few tricks!' said Dr Strait.
'Don't even think about it!' said Dr Susan.
'Well, I think the issue of consent is very relevant here,' said Dr Shorts. 'You must admit, Dai, that you only have to raise an eyebrow in the practice, and the staff will jump to it. Also, you say that you never need a chaperone with patients. Maybe it's the way you ask?'
'I didn't know I was such an ogre, but that reminds me: last week I asked a middle-aged woman, whom I've known since she was a teenager, if she wanted a chaperone. She said "Dr Strait – I reckon if you had wanted to take advantage of me, you'd have done it before now!"'
'I do find that picture disturbing, though,' said Dr Susan. 'I keep telling myself that it was done nearly 40 years ago and that times change, but I wonder how that kind of image would be received in the present climate, especially by an artist who is not established.'
'I suppose the artist was trying to disturb us,' said Dr Shorts. 'It's not as though there's a shortage of shocking images in contemporary art, but children are different – I suppose because they aren't able to give proper consent.'
'Perhaps artists just don't see it that way,' said Dr Strait. 'I get the impression that their art comes before everything else, even relationships.'
'That's why their lives are often such a mess,' said Dr Susan.

'Send for the social workers!' says Donald.
'And the mental handcuffs?' says Liam.

The next in our gallery of artists was also an important figure in his time.

John Singer Sargent (American: 1856–1925)

Google: enter 'John Singer Sargent Madame X' and click on 'images' – here is a whole range of variations of the painting, including studies.

John Singer Sargent was a society portraitist. He has been derided by many artists and critics because he fulfilled a traditional portraitist role within an art world increasingly dominated by the cutting edge of Modernism and Abstraction. A true artist was a law unto himself, not the servant of the wealthy elite said Modernists: art for art's sake.

Sargent began his career in earnest in Paris, but left following the disastrous reception of the portrait *Madame X* at the Salon of 1884. American Madame Gautreau had 'risen' from 'nothing'. Her scheming mother had managed to facilitate an advantageous marriage to a wealthy Parisian banker and ship owner. Sargent's portrait would, in the mother's eyes, confirm her daughter's newly achieved status once and for all.

Sargent himself was besotted with Madame Gautreau, going to enormous lengths to produce numerous preparatory studies. From his point of view, this was the portrait which was going to make his name, the Salon being the main forum for the launching of artists' reputations. But disaster struck. Instead of adulation the public response was tempestuous: the portrait was a caricature! Even before entering the building people outside were aware of the commotion within. Reviews referred to 'the ugliness of her profile' and 'the skin which is at the same time like that of a corpse and a clown'.[9] Sargent was instructed to remove the painting, by Madame Gautreau's mother. He refused, but nevertheless felt enough pressure to 'restore' the fallen dress strap (thus ruining the carefully constructed diagonal composition) and make the portrait less personal by re-titling it *Madame X*. Now nobody wanted *their* portrait done by *him.*

Such humiliating subservience to public taste made Sargent a good target for those in favour of the Modernist ideal that privileged the autonomy of the artist.

After several years of sustained effort this humiliating setback faced him with the possibility of total failure as an artist. He moved to London to 're-start' his career later that year.

Eventually Sargent recovered his position to the extent of becoming the most sought-after artist in London. Even so, he was reserved at social events, preferring to paint fashionable society rather than actually integrate with them. Instead he and his sister Emily formed a lifelong bond. One biographer has described her as the wife he never had.[10]

'Don't you say anything!' says Liam.
'Wouldn't dare!' says Donald.

Sargent was poor at verbal communication, especially at social gatherings: 'when he can't finish a sentence he waves his fingers before his face as a sort of signal for the conversation to go on without him'.[11] His total preoccupation with painting was recalled by his lifelong friend Vernon Lee:

'More and more it has seemed to me that Sargent's life was absorbed in his painting; and the summing up of the would-be biographer must, I think, be: *he painted*. To some of us he seemed occasionally to paint to the exclusion of living'.[11]

Suddenly, at the height of his popularity in 1907, Sargent announced 'No more *paughtraits*' (making fun of aristocratic pronunciation) ... I abhor and abjure them and hope never to do another, especially of the upper classes'.[12]

'Sounds like artistic burn-out?' said Dr Susan.
'But he must have made enough money to retire,' said Dr Strait.
'Burned out and loaded,' said Dr Shorts. 'A typical senior partner, don't you think?'
'I'm working on it,' said Dr Strait.

Frustrated would-be clients had to make do with quick charcoal sketches which Sargent himself disparagingly called 'mugshots'. It's interesting to note that the very medium is 'burnt out': grey/black in place of previous ravishing colour.

'He was lucky that his portrait work appealed to rich clients,' said Dr Shorts, 'because you get the strong impression that he didn't compromise.'
'Take it or leave it?' said Dr Susan.
'I find it difficult to communicate with words, when I'm tired,' said Dr Strait. 'So I tend to resort to gestures, too.'
'But it sounds to me as though Sargent's real communication was through his painting,' said Dr Shorts, 'and words, for him, were a second language at best.'

Hold onto that idea of paint language, guys. We shall return to it in another session (*see* Chapter 7). In the meantime, let's meet another painter who wasn't into compromise.

Rembradt van Rijn (Dutch: 1606–1669)

1 www.nationalgallery.org.uk (accessed 29.1.06)
   Click on 'Collection'.
   Click on 'Full Collection Index'.
   In 'Search' type 'Rembrandt' which brings up ten Rembrandts in the National Gallery, London.
2 For *The Anatomy Lesson of Dr Tulp* 1632: Google: type in 'Rembrandt Anatomy Lesson' and click on 'images'

3 For *Judas Returning the Pieces of Silver* 1629: Google: type in 'Rembrandt Judas returning silver' and click on 'images'.
4 Google: type in 'Rembrandt Rijksmuseum' which takes you to the Late Rembrandt room. Click on 'images' to get larger versions, e.g. *The Jewish Bride* 1669.

Rembrandt began studying painting under a mediocre artist, Jacob van Swanenburgh, for three years. More decisive for his development, however, were six months with the painter Pieter Lastman (c.1624) at Amsterdam. Rembrandt then set up as an independent artist in Leiden from c.1625–1631. Most of his output was biblical/history painting. As early as 1630 Rembrandt was attracting attention – the established artist and critic Constantin Huygens wrote a glowing account of *Judas Returning the Pieces of Silver* (1629, Lady Normanby Collection) admiring Judas' anguished facial expression and gestures.

His paintings from this time are usually small and meticulously finished. This is what patrons were used to and supported. However, even at this early stage there is the odd *impasto* and innovations such as *scraffito* with the butt end of a brush in wet paint.

'Impasto – sounds like the starter at our local trattoria!' says Donald.
'Means thick paint, slapped on,' says Liam.
'More like lasagne?' says Donald.
'If you say so,' says Liam.

Rembrandt moved to Amsterdam about 1631. His reputation was immediately assured by *The Anatomy Lesson of Dr Tulp* (1632).

For a decade he was Amsterdam's leading portraitist. This early success enabled him to collect significant works of art, and in 1639 he moved to a grand house in Amsterdam. However, he was already beginning to live rather flamboyantly for an artist, even a successful one.

In 1634 he married Saskia van Uylenburch, who was from an affluent family and came with a sizable dowry. Tragedy entered Rembrandt's life as three of their children died in infancy. Titus (1641–1668), the fourth, survived, but Saskia died shortly after he was born. He took a housekeeper, Hendrijke Stoffels, (1645) who became his common-law wife. Their daughter Cornelis was born in 1654.

Many masterpieces can be located within Rembrandt's biography, but more importantly for our purpose is that his painting style developed massively and independently over the decades. It is easy to appreciate now, thanks to modern art which has championed *the idea*, originality, individuality and art-for-art's-sake. However, his increasingly 'unfinished' painting style became unsaleable in his own time. Increasingly Rembrandt painted for himself, not the market – there's a palpable forward compulsion there. Meanwhile a number of his pupils left and, pleasing the art market, were financially more successful than their master.

The change in style is probably the main reason why Rembrandt became bankrupt in 1656. The other was his insatiable desire to collect beautiful objects which he used as props in his paintings. Armour, jewellery, furs and fabric filled his house. Such things don't come cheap.

'Like a kleptomaniac?' says Donald.
'Except that he didn't steal them,' says Liam.

Already acquainted with grief, his last years brought further tragedy – Hendrijke died in 1663 and Titus in 1668. Amazingly, far from crushing creativity, some of Rembrandt's most majestic works were painted shortly before his death, such as *The Jewish Bride* (1669, Rijksmuseum, Amsterdam).

The famous late self-portraits say it all: prolonged struggle, suffering, hardship, disillusionment and aloneness, but self-belief as a painter remains undiminished.

No one has ever painted themselves as Rembrandt did, before or since. Few artists can compete for more words written about them. How is it that a bankrupt from seventeenth-century Amsterdam still speaks so poignantly to so many today?

Dr Strait suddenly remembered how he had been stopped in his tracks by Rembrandt's eyes in the National Gallery last Sunday, as he waited to meet his 20-year-old daughter. He had been wandering through the galleries, past a row of Rembrandts he hadn't seen for years. A sudden rush of recognition had engulfed him as he sat down to contemplate Self Portrait at the age of 63 (1669).

'Here is one who feels as I do,' he had thought. 'I've never made an examination of my own face like that. It articulates the passing of time so painfully when compared with the painting over there – Self Portrait at the Age of 34, 1640. In that one he's doing well for himself – confident and wearing expensive clothes whilst proving his formidable skill to prospective patrons ... I'm not bankrupt, so why is it that the beaten Rembrandt speaks to me?'

He had moved close to the painting. The paint of the weary skin had looked clotted and agitated, re-visited many times over. There seemed a strange juxtaposition between this changeable, feelingful search for something through the paint and the assuredness of Rembrandt's pose. Passages of the painting varied enormously in thickness and texture.

'Why did he worry his paint so? What was he after?' Dr Strait had been struck by a feeling of searching and discovery.

He had resumed his seat, perplexed that the bankrupt from another country over three hundred years ago was somehow comforting to behold. It was only an object on a wall. But the oil bound in pigment, laid on canvas, had spoken in the quiet of the National Gallery, addressing a profound private need. No longer lonely at that moment, Dr Strait had felt nourished by contact with a fellow traveller through life, one who had trodden similar paths.

'That is so sad,' said Dr Susan.

'It makes sense of those self-portraits, though,' said Dr Shorts.

'Comes from being too high and mighty,' said Dr Strait. 'At least that Sargent fellow knew which side his bread was buttered, whatever he said at the end.'

'You see patients like that, don't you?' said Dr Shorts. 'They don't seem to be able to manage relationships with the world, and they don't learn, even though they keep coming off worst.'

'It wasn't his fault that his wife and children died,' said Dr Susan, 'and he must have made relationships with Saskia and Hendrijke.'

Yes, I agree. Lay off him, chaps! If you had been able to send Rembrandt to be straightened out by some therapist, would we have had the developments in his work that inspire modern artists and speak so eloquently to us in the twenty-first century?

In contrast, the next painter in our gallery was successful throughout his life. 'He must have given the patrons what they wanted,' said Dr Strait.

Sir Peter Paul Rubens (Dutch: 1577–1640)

Google: type 'Rubens Three Graces Prado' and click on 'images'.

Rubens only learnt local painting traditions from mediocre local painters. But meanwhile he acquired a thorough knowledge of the classics, Latin, and the major European languages which set him in good stead for his future life. As well as being one of the greatest artists of his time, Rubens was also an important diplomat, scholar and businessman – in short, a seventeenth-century polymath. In 1598 he became a Master of the Guild of St. Luke in Antwerp.

'Business studies,' said Dr Strait. 'That's what these artists need.'

Two years later Rubens went to Italy which is where he really developed his artistic education. He lived in Rome until 1602. In 1603, on behalf of Vincenzo Gonzaga, Duke of Mantua, he went to Spain where he painted the equestrian portrait of the Duke of Lerma. He also made copies after Titian. In 1604 Rubens returned to Mantua, in the service of Gonzaga. In the years 1605–1608 he lived in Genoa and Rome as a portraitist of the upper classes. Still driven by his personal quest to learn, Rubens made copies of Michelangelo's sculptures and frescoes. He also worked from Titian, Tintoretto and Correggio.

'It shows amazing persistence and determination,' said Dr Shorts, 'to spend all that time learning by copying the old masters.'

'Ah, but he had put himself in a position financially to be able to do it,' said Dr Strait.

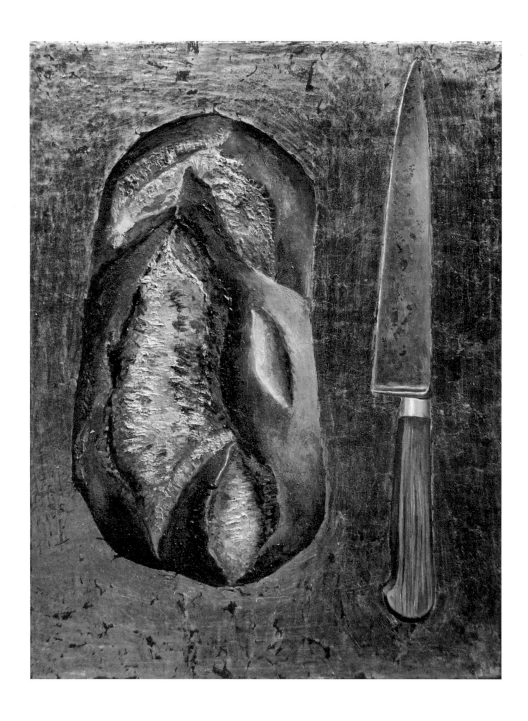

Plate 1: Our Daily Bread (2005) (private collection, Britain)

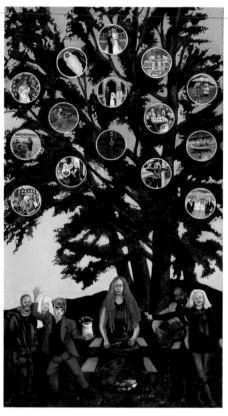

Plate 2: Tree of Life I (2003) (collection of the artist)

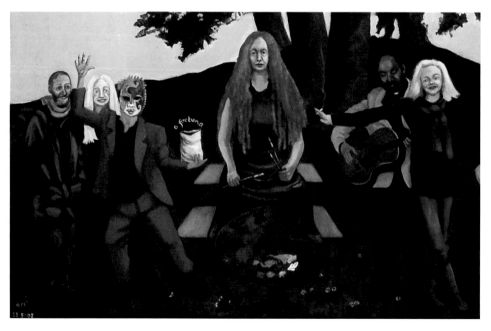

Plate 3: Detail of Plate 2   (figures)

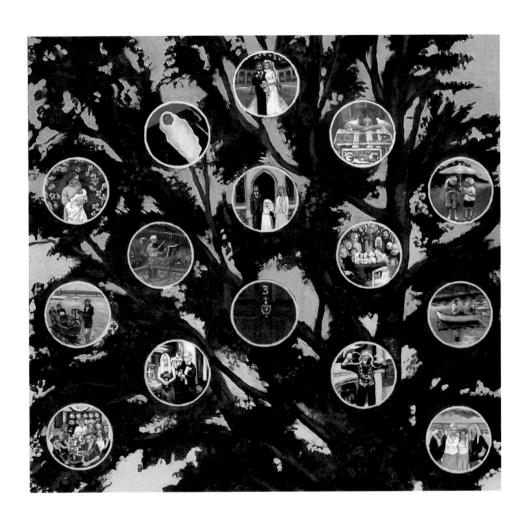

Plate 4: Detail of Plate 2 (roundels)

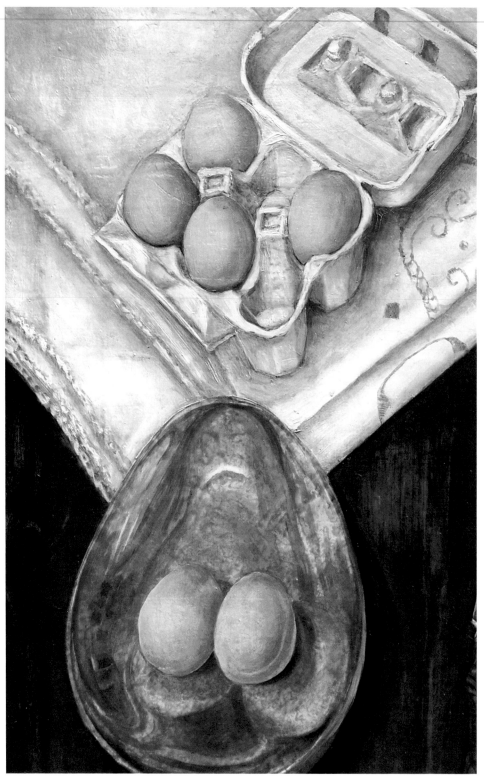
Plate 5: Scramble (1998) (private collection, Britain)

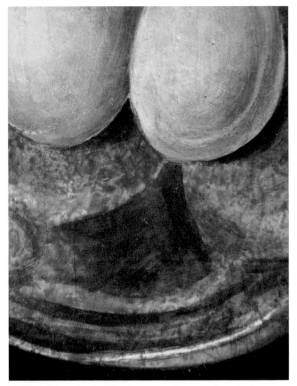

Plate 6: Detail of Plate 5

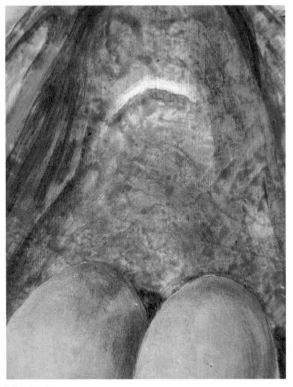

Plate 7: Detail of Plate 5

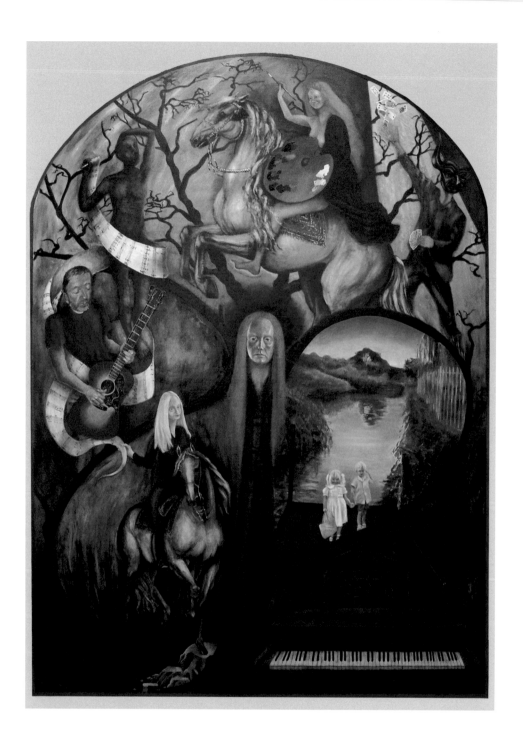

Plate 8: Tree of Life II (2004) (collection of the artist)

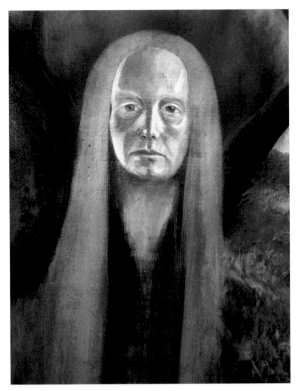

Plate 9: Detail of Plate 8 (self portrait)

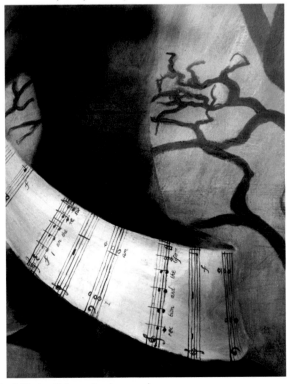

Plate 10: Detail of Plate 8 (musical score)

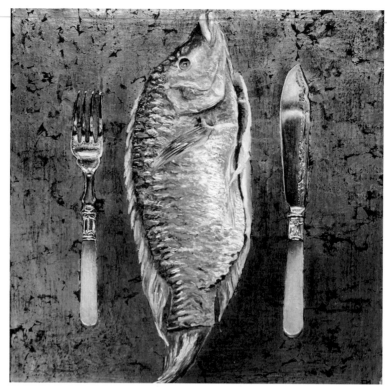

Plate 11: Fish for Dinner (2005) (private collection, United Arab Emirates)

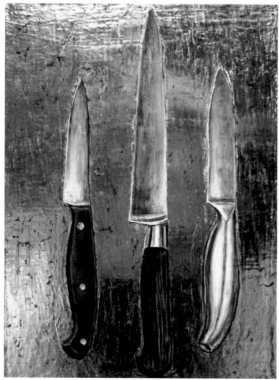

Plate 12: Knife Trio (2005) (collection of the artist)

In 1608 he returned to Antwerp. Although the city had lost its position as a powerful international centre of trade, it had become the cultural headquarters of the Counter-Reformation in Flanders – a Flanders dominated by Spain. It was a good place for a painter because the Church and the Court of Brussels supported the arts. Rubens immediately became the leading painter of Antwerp, an inevitability given his immense talent, drive, education and social standing.

'No flies on this chap!' said Dr Strait.

In 1609 he was appointed painter to the Archduke Albert of Austria and his wife, the Viceroys for the King of Spain. In the same year he married.

Between 1609 and 1621 Rubens undertook an astonishing number of major commissions. His studio, adjoined to his prestigious house in Antwerp, is a very grand three-storey building where a 'factory production line' of employed painters facilitated this prodigious output. Basically, the more prestigious the patron and/or they more they paid, the more the master's own hand touched the commissioned work. This is a far cry from the stereotypical artist starving in his garret, as illustrated by Rubens' statement: 'I regard all the world as my country, and I believe I should be very welcome everywhere'.[6] This was not an exaggeration – when he went to Spain on a political mission in 1628 he so charmed Philip IV that many portraits and other paintings were immediately commissioned. By the time of his death over a hundred Rubens' paintings were in Spanish palaces. In 1629 he visited London in the dual role of diplomat and painter, whereupon Charles I was so enthralled that he knighted Rubens. What was it that made Rubens' painting so attractive? The bottom line, so to speak, is the way he painted flesh. The voluptuous sensuous excesses of a bottom, breast or thigh contain the most expressive unanticipated colour and painterly touch. He articulates on the patron's behalf, as it were (*see* chapter 7 on paint language).

The death of his first wife in 1626, affected Rubens deeply: 'I have no pretensions about ever attaining a stoic equanimity.'[6] However, in 1630 he married the 16-year-old Helene Fourment. She was the epitome of all his models and her likeness appears throughout his late work, often as a saint or deity, for example the left-hand figure in *The Three Graces* (1636–40).

'Do you realise he was 53!' said Dr Strait.
'There's hope for you yet, Dai!' said Dr Shorts.
'That's the middle-aged man's fantasy,' said Dr Susan. 'The trouble is that some of
    my patients try to live it out, usually with devastating effects to themselves and
    those connected with them.'
'You mean leaving their wives?' said Dr Shorts.
'And children,' said Dr Susan.

At the end of his life, Rubens retired from public life, but not from painting. The wealthy artist bought a manorial residence with land to the south of Antwerp, called *Het Steen.* Here he painted a number of panoramic landscapes from the grounds, of varying sizes from small to huge, and at varying times of day, including nocturnes. He was painting for himself, and these canvases display an avant-garde freedom of colour, brushwork and emotional response. Rubens was celebrating the country he loved.

'That's the way to do it,' said Dr Strait. 'Don't waste time on things nobody wants – at least until you're so well off that you don't have to care.'
'Very level-headed, I'm sure,' said Dr Shorts, 'but it doesn't usually go with the artistic temperament, does it?'
'What about Tracey Emin and Damien Hirst, and all those people hanging onto Saatchi's coat tails?' said Dr Susan.
'But what about poor old Rembrandt, and Van Gogh?' said Dr Shorts.

Not forgetting another tragic figure, guys.

'Oh no, not him!' says Donald.

Mark Rothko (American: 1903–1970)

Google: type 'Rothko classic paintings' or 'Rothko Tate Modern' and click on 'images'.

Rothko was one of the leading figures of American Abstract Expressionism.

'Abstract gobbledegook!' says Donald.
'Calm down,' says Liam. 'It just means expressing strong emotions through abstract works.'
'You may like to wallow in emotions,' says Donald, 'but I just want to be somewhere else fast!'
'Not that you were at all emotional about that goal they scored against you!' says Liam.

Rothko came to the USA in 1913 as a Russian Jewish immigrant, knowing no English. Despite this, he won a scholarship for Yale. His daughter feels that the decision to become a painter was a philosophical one, post-Yale. He moved toward abstraction during the 1940s and founded an art school with a number of his peers in New York. His aim, and that of his art school, was the search for the simplest means with which to express universal truths. His mature work developed from around 1950. This is characterised by large rectangular bands of colour (often thin washes of different hues) arranged parallel to each other, usually in a vertical format.

'Goal posts!' says Donald

The edges of these shapes are softly uneven, giving them a hazy, pulsating quality, as if they are floating on the canvas. The background colours subtly yet dramatically relate to the colour of these rectangles. Often the paintings are enormous, and their effect often encourages calmness and contemplation in the viewer. They can be understood in terms of symbols presented through colour, line and shape.

'Symbols? says Donald.
'Goal posts, doorways, containers? Who knows?' says Liam.

As a personality, Rothko was introspective and proud. In terms of outward events in his life, there is little to tell. He refused to join group exhibitions and controlled those who wrote about him, offending a number of established art critics along the way.

The Seagram Murals (*see* chapter 1) arrived, as a gift, at The Tate on 22 February 1970. On this very day Rothko committed suicide in his studio. He was 66 and had been depressed for some time. Two years earlier he had suffered an aneurism which left him severely weakened and on heavy medication. Also he was a heavy drinker. The autopsy cited a drug overdose and slit wrists.

'Now you understand why I had to get away from that room at Tate Modern!' says
*   Donald. 'I felt really depressed!'*
'You were in touch with your feelings,' says Liam.
'Not mine – his!'
'Maybe so – but if it's true, it's even more amazing,' says Liam, 'that a painting can put
*   a person like you in touch with another's feelings.'*

'Depression always seems an inadequate word for it,' said Dr Strait. 'That's what
    William Styron says in *Darkness Visible* – you may have seen it on my shelf'.[13]
'Not the most inviting title,' said Dr Shorts.
'He's a Pulitzer prize-winning novelist writing about his own depression,' said
    Dr Strait, 'which he describes as more like a brainstorm so intense that you'll do
    anything to get away from it.'
'Including suicide?' said Dr Susan.
'Judging whether life is or is not worth living amounts to answering the funda-
    mental question of philosophy,' said Dr Strait.
'Who's saying that?' said Dr Shorts.
'It's Styron quoting Camus,' said Dr Strait, 'but it's an interesting question.'
'Maybe Rothko was asking himself that question over and over again in his
    murals,' said Dr Susan. 'It might account for the very different reactions that
    people have to them.'
'Doorways to what exactly?' said Dr Shorts. 'There's the ambiguity.'
'Emptiness or infinity?' said Dr Strait. 'We Celts understand about that.'
'Do you think you have ever prevented a suicide?' said Dr Shorts.
'I'm sure I have – quite a number of times,' said Dr Strait. 'People need to be told
    that they can get better, because it's hard for them to believe that, when they're
    at the bottom of the pit. Styron says it was true for him, too.'
'Are you all right, Dai?' said Dr Susan.
'I'm not suicidal, if that's what you mean,' said Dr Strait.

'It's hard picking up the pieces afterwards,' said Dr Shorts. 'The effect on families is devastating.'

'And long-lasting,' said Dr Susan. 'I try to help them to understand that it is an illness, and that their relative wasn't responsible for his or her actions.'

'Do they believe it?' said Dr Strait.

'I find it helpful to explain that perception is altered, in severe depression, so that the patient's dark thoughts seem logical. It's as though they are making a rational decision for the good of themselves and everyone else.'

'And what does your religion say about it?' said Dr Strait. 'Do they go to hell?'

'I don't know if I believe in the traditional idea of hell.'

'It's a problem for some people with religious beliefs,' said Dr Strait. 'At least, I've found it so.'

'Well, I can't believe that God would reject a person who was seriously ill,' said Dr Susan. 'Anyway, who knows the state of another's mind at the point of death?'

At which point, I feel I should call the meeting to order. We seem to have come a long way, at least emotionally, by reflecting on the stories about artists (though we have strayed a little into painting and meaning, and also into paint language, both of which are the subjects of future sessions). Admittedly, the stories have been sketchy, even fragmentary. There has been so much written about these people, but I will leave it up to you to decide whether to find out more.

I think we were trying to gain insight into the meaning of paintings, that don't necessarily contain a story, by looking at the painters themselves. The main thing to recognise is that *behind every painting is another person*. Perhaps it's like looking behind the façade of a patient who comes to your surgery? All you have are your own reactions to what they are presenting. *You have to look inside yourself*, in order to begin to understand someone else. What you were doing tonight was projecting your own feelings about the artists' stories and, in the end, it's all you can do. It's what Sartre called *anguish*, the notion that none of us knows about the world or other people except through our own internal perception.[14] Maybe, but I think that it's good enough.

For more on Rothko's paintings, *see* Chapter 6.

References

1   Watt G (2005) Frida Kahlo. *Br J Gen Pract*. **55**: 646–7

2   Herrera H (1972) *Frida: a biography of Frida Kahlo*. Harper and Row, New York.

3   Fuentes C (1998) *The Diary of Frida Kahlo: an intimate self-portrait*. Abradale Books, New York.

4   Greer G (2005) The Culture Show. BBC2.

5   Sandblom P (1997) *Creativity and Disease: how illness affects literature, art and music*. Marion Boyars, London.

6 Osborne H (ed) (1970) *The Oxford Companion to Art*. Clarendon Press, Oxford.

7 Metzger IF and Walther R (1999) *Van Gogh*. Taschen, Köln.

8 Lampert C (1993) *Lucien Freud: recent work*. Whitechapel Art Gallery, London.

9 Josephin P (1998) Le Salon de 1884. *L'Artiste*. **54**(1): 441.

10 Kilmurray E and Ormond R (1998) *John Singer Sargent*. Tate Gallery Publishing, London.

11 Olson S (1986) *John Singer Sargent: his portrait*. Macmillan London Limited, London.

12 Hills P (1978) *John Singer Sargent*. Whiteny Museum of Art, New York.

13 Styron W (1991) *Darkness Visible: a memoir of madness*. Jonathan Cape, London.

14 Sartre J-P (1957) *Being and Nothingness* (trans. Barnes HE). Methuen, London.

Resource

Ideas for the section on John Singer Sargent were drawn from:

- Middleton E (2000) *Artistic Integrity and Patronage in two portraits by John Singer Sargent* (MA dissertation). University of Nottingham. Unpublished.

CHAPTER 6

Painting and meaning

Paintings are a vehicle for expressing emotions rather than using words, but the messages are often ambiguous and operate on different levels. Individuals respond in different ways that are valid for them. Being prepared to look inside oneself, without fear, may help to understand the artist's and our patients' standpoints, and help them to be recognised. In doing so, we must face fundamental issues, such as loss, mortality and belief.

'I've been thinking about Rothko,' says Liam.
'Something told me that we hadn't heard the last of him!' says Donald.
'It's fascinating that I feel just the opposite way from you when I sit and look at those paintings,' says Liam. 'I feel tranquil, as though I'm contemplating infinity.'
'Or nothing!' says Donald. 'No, it's worse than that − more like a negative force.'
'The dark side?' says Liam.
'You've been watching too much science fiction!' says Donald.

Mark Rothko said: 'The progression of a painter's work . . . will be toward clarity; toward the elimination of all obstacles between the painter and the idea, and between the idea and the observer . . . to achieve this clarity is, inevitably, to be understood'.[1]

'Why didn't he write the idea down, if he thought it was so important to communicate it?' said Dr Strait.
'Maybe because it wasn't an idea that could be put in words, at least not by him,' said Dr Shorts.
'It's as though he feels that his idea comes from outside himself,' said Dr Susan, 'that it's part of a common consciousness, not just in his own head.'
'That's rubbish!' said Dr Strait.
'No, it's not! I think he's imagining that there are ideas floating out there somewhere, with the painter and the observer on the ground − and their vision is obscured by a kind of cloud. He sees it as the painter's job to brush away the cloud, by the way he does the brushstrokes.'
'That's a very poetic concept,' said Dr Shorts.
'Thank you, Simon.'

Google: type in 'Rothko Tate Modern' and click on 'images'.
Alternative: repeat the above, but search under 'web' – this brings up the relevant page for Rothko from the Tate's artists index/collection.

His paintings are vast, usually dark canvases. They operate on more than one level, but the first thing that affects you is their size – around three metres high on average. They envelop you. In an interview (1951), Rothko explained this choice of scale: 'You are in it; it isn't something you command'.[2] He was asked how far from the paintings an observer should stand – 'eighteen inches'.[3] Rothko explains further: 'I paint very large pictures. I realise that historically the function of painting large pictures is painting something very grandiose and pompous. The reason I paint them, however . . . is precisely because I want to be very intimate and human'.[1]

Elkins tells us that Rothko is giving us, in the most profound and general sense, an image of what loss and mortality look like, yet at the same time these massive canvases are experienced by some viewers as strangely transcendental.[2] The blank rectangles within the dark canvases have been likened to panoramic land-scapes (horizontal lines equating with horizons), or alternatively 'landscapes of the spirit', monumental classical architecture or grave-like spaces.

'I can see how those images could induce a transcendental state,' said Dr Susan. 'It might feel as though you are going out of yourself and being absorbed into the universe.'
'Or going into the grave and ceasing to exist,' said Dr Strait.
'If you're depressed, it might make you feel like that,' said Dr Susan.
'Nothing wrong with me!' said Dr Strait.
'Loss and mortality are important issues for our patients, whatever their beliefs, and whatever our beliefs,' said Dr Shorts. 'Your Mr Choleric, Dai – he's angry because he's losing his health and his status. My Mr Tidy – he's worried about his mortality. I'm not sure about Mrs Liszt – something's going on, but it's hard to interpret the signals.'
'Like a painting,' said Dr Susan. 'It's hard to interpret the paint language!'
'I can save you a lot of trouble with Rothko's message,' said Dr Strait. 'There's nothing out there – when you're dead, it's finished!'
'Not much comfort in that,' said Dr Shorts.
'We all know what your views are, Dai, and you're entitled to them, said Dr Susan, 'but somehow I don't think that Rothko was an atheist, even though he committed suicide.'
'Neither of you really know – that's the point,' said Dr Shorts. 'the images are ambiguous and people interpret them individually.'

To Elkins, sitting in the Rothko Chapel, Houston, Texas, experiencing the huge empty black canvases felt: 'a little dangerous, like playing at drowning'.[2] For him: 'the really unendurable fact is that meaning is what's absent, and people who intellectualise Rothko use history and philosophy as a balm that soothes the nameless loss'.[2]

---

www.rothkochapel.org
Google: type 'Rothko Chapel Houston' and click on 'images'.

'There you are,' said Dr Strait. 'No meaning – I told you so!'
'I can see that it's difficult, or impossible to translate images like that into words,' said Dr Shorts, 'but you can't necessarily interpret them as the artist saying that existence is meaningless. Perhaps the meaning is in the paint itself – the feelings it induces in us; the feelings of the artist. We have no way of knowing if they are similar.'
'Hence the ambiguity,' said Dr Susan.

James Elkins writes at some length, with a painter's perception and understanding, about Rothko. He cites a number of personal responses to experiencing Rothko's huge empty black canvases in the visitors' books. Since 1972, when the chapel was dedicated, around 5000 comments have been entered.

- 'Probably the most moving experience I have had with art.'
- 'Once more I am moved – to tears.'
- 'This makes me fall down.'
- 'A religious experience that moves one to tears.'
- 'I wish I could cry.'[2]

The 'meaning' of an artwork depends partly on the observer, who approaches it from an individual standpoint in time, with an individual personality, history and experience. The received meaning of the artwork is valid for the individual observer. The artist interacts with and absorbs ideas from the outside world. He then communicates with his inner world and, as it were, pulls up a bucket containing ideas and feelings that are a product of the interaction between the two sources of inspiration, that is, his inner and outer worlds. The resulting art work is experienced by another person, and interacts with their own inner/outer worlds. Perception, by both the artist and observer, is coloured by individual experience – and inner worlds. To fully interact with a work of art, the observer must also 'pull up a bucket' from within their own depths.

The experience is not always positive, but there is usually potential for learning. As we have seen, art can be disturbing – either because there is conflict with the observer's values and beliefs, or because the message resonates only too well with experiences that have been denied and buried in the recesses of the psyche. The resulting dissonance can be dealt with by erecting further barriers of denial, or learning by integrating the new experience into ourselves.

'I haven't changed my point of view,' said Dr Strait, 'but I think I have learnt something about ambiguity and paintings.'

Elkins states that Rothko: 'wanted to make religious art', and quotes Rothko himself as saying in an interview in 1957: 'The people who weep before my pictures are having the same religious experience I had when I painted them'.[2] Rothko continues: 'I'm interested only in expressing basic human emotions; tragedy, ecstasy, doom, and so on – and the fact that lots of people break down and cry when confronted with my pictures shows that I *communicate* those basic human emotions'.[2]

'That makes more sense,' said Dr Shorts. 'I think emotions are what his pictures communicate, rather than ideas as he seemed to be saying earlier.'
'Yes, and he also seems to be saying that experience of the basic emotions is similar for everyone,' said Dr Susan.
'Debatable, I'd say,' said Dr Strait. 'Some people seem to feel things more deeply than others.'
'They're called artists!' said Dr Shorts.
'Somebody had a theory about the *collective unconscious*,' said Dr Susan.
'It was Jung – and it's rubbish!' said Dr Strait.

'Collective unconscious?' says Donald. 'Sounds like Nottingham as the clubs are closing!'
'That's not as far off as you might think,' says Liam. 'I think it just means that we each have an inherited common influence on our psyche from the physical structure of the central nervous system.'
'The lowest common denominator?' says Donald.
'A bit like the id,' says Liam.
'If you say so!' says Donald.

However, artists and art are often not straightforward. Rothko is also quoted as saying 10 years later: 'My relation with God was not very good and it has gotten worse day by day. I started out thinking the paintings should have a religious subject matter, but they became dark, on their own'.[2] In support of this ambiguity, Rothko's biographer, James Breslin is quoted as saying: 'when Rothko wasn't urging the religious import of his paintings he was denying the religious character imputed to them by others.'[3] For example he would say 'I am not a religious man.'

'Perhaps it depends what he meant by 'religious',' said Dr Susan.
'It's not difficult to recognise religion when I see it a hundred miles away!' said Dr Strait.
'Keep your hair on, Dai!' said Dr Shorts. 'Maybe he identified the word 'religious' with ritual?'
'You mean organised religion?'
'Yes, as opposed to private spirituality.'
'I'm not sure I accept that as a concept either,' said Dr Strait.

Bronowski said that the difference between science and art is that science is always attempting to distinguish between 'x' and 'not x' (testing a hypothesis), whereas they often co-exist in a work of art, that is 'x' and 'not x' at the same time.[4]

'Like Janus,' says Liam.
'Didn't he used to play for Newcastle?' says Donald.
'Roman God – with two heads,' says Liam.

Opposite sides of the coin, like hope and despair, can be presented simultaneously. This might help to explain the variety of reactions to Rothko's landscapes, and the ambiguity of his own 'explanations'. Ambiguity can be what art is about, and this in turn can reflect human nature.

Perhaps Sigmund Freud (grandfather of Lucien the painter) can help us at this point. He started out as a respectable medical scientist – a neurologist. As a result of his clinical work he became interested in *conversion hysteria*, where patients appeared to produce physical symptoms because of psychological hang ups.[5] These days we might call them *somatisers*. Freud came to the conclusion that patients like this were denying disturbing psychological material and pushing it down into the unconscious. This was effective, but the psychic energy associated with the repressed material was continually seeking release by physical expression, and thus giving rise to the symptoms. Initially, Freud tried to uncover the distressing material using hypnosis. Later, he developed the technique of *free association*, in which the patient was urged to express the first thought that offered itself and the train of that thought was subsequently explored. During this process, he frequently encountered *resistance*, which sometimes manifested itself by ambiguous or contradictory responses – a form of denial, he asserted. Thus he argued that the patients' responses could mean the opposite of what they were actually saying. So Freud was always right, because you could never disprove his conclusions; in other words they lacked *falsifiability*. This was the point at which he parted company with science.

Freud attempted to discover more about the unconscious part of the mind by analysing dreams, first of all his own.[6] He found that it was possible to access the material by writing it down immediately on waking from a dream. Otherwise most of them are forgotten very quickly. Often, he found that the *manifest content* made little sense, but that some parts were paradoxically associated with strong emotions. The next step was to use free association in relation to those parts, in order to arrive at the *latent content* of the dream. His conclusion was that the emotional content of dreams was the energy associated with repressed thoughts, and that these were often of a sexual nature. This gave him rather a bad name, and it got much worse when he extended these theories to include childhood sexual experiences. To be fair, he later admitted that he could have been mistaken in this area, but it was too late for many people.

In order to accommodate these discoveries, he proposed a model of the psyche with three components that have become very familiar to us: The *id* is the seat of unconscious desires which are constantly seeking release (the *pleasure principle*); the *super ego* is the conscience or internalised parent which is the source of our *life script*, that is – what we are expected to do; and the *ego* is the ringmaster that tries to keep equilibrium between the demands of the id, super ego and external reality. It remains a hypothetical model, without any connection to the physical structures of the brain, except that you might identify the id with the more primitive parts. Perhaps you would agree that man's behaviour could be seen as a product of animal urges and higher rationality. It gets a little confusing, because the *unconscious* appears to be involved in all of the three components (id, super ego and ego). Freud is not an easy read and he appears to change his mind frequently in his later writings.

He explained dreams as *wish fulfilment*. Repressed thoughts and experiences, and the urges of the id are able to overcome the censorship mechanism that usually operates efficiently during the day, by attaching their emotional energy to recent memory traces. The ego attempts to cobble them all together in a sequence, and the energy is released to the surface. Job done, you might think, but unfortunately the sources of this uncomfortable force do not dry up in a hurry, if ever. This is, perhaps, good news for private psychoanalysts, and it is also good for the production of art.

Dreams and creativity rely on a similar source of energy. The artist's perceptions of reality are like the recent memory traces, onto which the unconscious hitches a ride. He *puts down a bucket* into his inner self and makes use of psychic energy to animate a transformed vision in the resulting work of art. Usually this happens when he is awake – so you might draw the conclusion that artistic temperaments can more easily gain access to their unconscious: they have an enhanced facility to daydream. It could perhaps explain their frequent trait of instability, this constant exposure to what others repress. Artists create because of their inner drive: they *need* to do it.

Perhaps most of you don't feel the same need to look inside yourselves and unlock the volcanoes, but if you really want to understand art, think again. When you observe a work of art, perhaps focusing initially on narrative aspects, a superficial first impression is likely to give way to engagement with the emotional power behind the work, at least if the work is contemplated for any length of time. To relate to the emotion, you must also put down your buckets into your inner recesses. And all of a sudden, you are in contact with the raw power of another psyche, perhaps long dead, as manifested by the reaction in your own core. Is that scary or what? Of course, in the case of a painting, you can choose to move away.

'Very quickly, in your case!' says Liam.
'Don't remind me!' says Donald.

This conflict between the external, and perhaps superficial view of humanity, and the internal deeper perspective has also been played out in the field of Social Science. At one end of the scale, we have the behaviourists, who are interested in what is measurable – which amounts to external behaviour. Their legacy is reinforcement schedules – sticks and carrots. You might say that this is control without understanding. They might reply that it doesn't matter, since nothing apart from behaviour makes any difference, and because anything beyond behaviour cannot be known with any certainty.

On the other hand, advocates of the internal perspective would argue that the behaviourists have an impoverished view of humanity. Admittedly, reliance on what the subjects choose to tell them about their inner worlds is unscientific – just like Freud. The results of such investigations are questionable, but potentially richer in terms of understanding humanity. Moreover, a kind of validity can be achieved by using what they call overlapping perspectives – using a variety of approaches and methods, in the hope of finding considerable common ground.

'They could just be wrong over and over again,' said Dr Strait.

'But human beings are not robots,' said Dr Shorts. 'We have to try and understand what is going on inside. Otherwise we could send Messrs Choleric and Tidy down to a service centre!'

'And it sounds as though science is not much use to us in trying to achieve that kind of understanding,' said Dr Susan, 'but these paintings have really opened up a discussion about fundamental issues.'

'I know that Freud has his critics,' said Dr Shorts, 'but I really like the psychodynamic model. The opposing forces in the psyche, with the ego trying to hold it all together, and not always succeeding – it makes sense to me. Did I ever tell you – I once analysed some of my dreams?'

'Do we really need to go there?' said Dr Strait.

'Don't worry! I'm not going to tell you! But they were really horrible – and do you know – afterwards, I felt kind of free.'

'In what way?' said Dr Susan.

'Well, I thought: yes, I *am* an animal, with all sorts of urges that I couldn't talk about, but *so is everybody else*! And there's nothing to be ashamed of, just because my controller goes off-duty while I'm asleep, and all sorts of images and thoughts get mixed up together. When I wake up, I'm fully human again – rational and moral, at least most of the time.'

'Excuse me – I'm just off to bed with my little notebook!' said Dr Strait.

'It was a very brave and honest statement, and you shouldn't laugh,' said Dr Susan.

'Apart from the feeling of freedom,' said Dr Shorts, 'I found it helped me to be more tolerant of other people, knowing what lurks below the surface in all of us.'

'That's why you're such a soft touch, Simon!' said Dr Strait. 'I'll buy you a new cardigan for Christmas!'

'I don't think you're so hard-boiled as you make out,' said Dr Shorts. 'Anyway, you have to admit that we could get overwhelmed by the sheer mountain of misery that comes through the door. In the past, I've felt frustrated and angry over the way some people behave towards each other, and us. Sometimes I still do, but now I can often see life more indulgently.'

'Like *Vanity Fair?*' said Dr Strait.

'Yes, the circus goes on and we can't change it, even if we impact a little on individuals here and there.'

'But those individuals are important, each one of them,' said Dr Susan.

I don't like to interrupt this interesting discussion, but I would like to move on. Freedom is an idea that was particularly important for our second artist of the evening

Following the Second World War, interest in *Existentialism* was fuelled by the writings of Jean Paul Sartre. His belief was that the cost of the new post-war freedom from traditional values and beliefs, was that of isolation.

Francis Bacon voiced existentialist views when he stated 'man now realises that he is an accident, that he is a completely futile being'[7] and his paintings reflect this belief. Layers of meaning contribute to Bacon's imagery. Take, for example, his series of screaming Popes which he began in the mid-1950s (www.francis-bacon.cx/themes/the_popes.html).

We need to consider memory – Bacon's early experiences of sexual abuse and subsequent homosexual lifestyle, his aggressively dominant father. Visual imagery also plays a part – the 'still' of the screaming nurse in Eisenstein's film *The Battleship Potemkin*, Velazquez's *Pope Innocent X* (Galerie Doria Pamphili, Rome) and the detail of the woman screaming in Poussin's *Massacres of the Holy Innocents* (c.1650, Musee Conde, Chantilly, France). Bacon had also got hold of a book on diseases of the mouth which he found compelling, declaring that he would like to paint the mouth as expressively as Monet painted sunsets. Personal witness also came into the screaming Popes series. Bacon said, 'I've always been very moved by pictures about slaughterhouses ... animals just being taken up before they were slaughtered ... they're so aware of what is going to happen to them'.[7] Media footage also played a part such as the recent Nuremberg Trials (1945–1949), in which some individuals were placed in bulletproof glass boxes. Where is Christianity in all this? It's a Pope each time who is screaming. Is he victim or aggressor? Bacon's series is a heady mix of ambiguity, memory, disgust and visually stimulating imagery. His imagery usually comprises a lone distorted, often disturbing figure set in an enclosed interior space. Bacon wanted to be able to 'open up or rather, should I say, unlock the valves of feeling and therefore return the onlooker to life more violently.'[7]

'What did you say, Donald?'
'I said come back, Rothko – all is forgiven!'

'That stuff you were just talking about, Simon,' said Dr Strait. 'This Bacon chap has brought it all up to the surface!'

'I would have been more shocked by it before,' said Dr Shorts.

'I don't think man is a futile being,' said Dr Susan.

'Of course – you're a Christian!' said Dr Strait.

'But I'm not a Roman Catholic,' said Dr Susan, 'so I'm not at all offended by Popes in cages. I just think that he was very angry with his father ... with God the Father!'

'For making such a mess of the world!' said Dr Strait.

'His paintings are certainly full of cruelty and suffering,' said Dr Shorts.

'It's not surprising, and I feel very sorry for him!' said Dr Susan.

'You don't need to – he's dead!' said Dr Strait.

'But death isn't the end,' said Dr Susan.

'How do you know that?' said Dr Strait. 'Don't tell me – it's your faith!'

'Hang on!' said Dr Shorts. 'It seems to me that both of you are speaking from a position of belief. You are intelligent people, along with thousands of others who hold opposing views on the question.'

'I'm speaking from a position of unbelief!' said Dr Strait.

'You believe that there is no God,' said Dr Shorts. 'You can't prove that you're right, any more than Susan can. Myself, I reserve judgement. There are arguments for and against. Some days, different arguments seem more convincing. At least it's a rational position.'

'But human rationality is limited,' said Dr Susan. 'We can classify things and discover the relationships between them, but we can't begin to understand their origins nor the nature of infinity.'

'There's no need to understand these things,' said Dr Strait. 'We exist and will soon cease to exist, and the world is going the same way. It's a waste of time to look for a reason when there is none.'

'It's human nature to try and understand things,' said Dr Shorts, 'but there's always another frontier behind each bit of scientific progress. Even so, it's amazing to contemplate how much we do know: right from the 'big bang' to the evolution of life on earth, and of course ourselves, through to the accelerating expansion of the known universe.'

'Do you not think that the so-called 'big bang' is evidence of God's hand, unfolding his creation?' said Dr Susan.

'The short answer is no!' said Dr Strait.

'Well it seems a strange thing to me,' said Dr Shorts, 'that here we are, apparently alone in this vast universe, with our thought bubbles. Did you see Dennis Potter's last television play *Cold Lazarus?*'

'He died before it was shown,' said Dr Strait.

'Yes, very ironic,' said Dr Shorts. 'They preserved this man's head, and found a way to reanimate the brain by an infusion of neuropeptides, or some rubbish like that. Anyway, they had the head wired up to a television set, so that they could enter his thoughts by way of a sound and light show – don't scoff; I'm sure Dennis was having a good laugh writing it!'

'I remember now,' said Dr Strait. 'It was just like a thought bubble expanding, when the television burst into life!'

'And they were using his experiences as worldwide entertainment in order to fund the scientific development – even watching football matches that he'd been to,' said Dr Shorts. 'Completely ridiculous, but then I thought *where does the bubble of consciousness come from?*'

'It's the soul,' said Dr Susan.

'Perhaps you're right,' said Dr Shorts. 'Surely you don't think, Dai, that this light and sound and feelings show that we have is just a product of neurological feedback loops, however complex?'

'Why not?' said Dr Strait.

'Because it's the presence of our self-awareness – the whole experience of being here. I can't make a connection between that and lumps of tissue.'

'Perhaps you just don't know enough,' said Dr Strait, 'but what's the point of all this speculation?'

'Well, I find that I'm confronted by the issue of mortality,' said Dr Shorts. 'Even if I want to hide from it, my patients keep reminding me.'

'By dying?' said Dr Susan.

'More by the questions they keep putting to me, without actually asking the question, if you know what I mean.'

'I know,' said Dr Strait.

'So, do you think that we should take the bull by the horns and talk to them about these issues?' said Dr Susan.

'Not necessarily. I mean you have to be careful not to use your professional position to promote your own beliefs.'

'You have to respect their position,' said Dr Strait.

'Yes, and that means being led by them.'

'And being careful how you respond,' said Dr Strait.

'Of course, yes. But what I really meant was to be at ease with yourself about these things, as far as you can be. Then you can be ready for anything. You can look them in the eye *and not be afraid*. I think that's what people need. Even if you are afraid, I still think it helps people to know that you're there, and not running away.'

'Are you afraid, Simon?' said Dr Susan.

'Yes sometimes, but then I thought 'let's unpick this fear'. If existence finishes with death, it won't be my problem. A few close friends and family will be upset, but they'll get over it. If I had warning it was going to happen, I could have regrets about all the events in my family that I'll never see, but it's not very logical. It would be better to concentrate on the way I live now, so that they would have good memories of me.'

'And if there is something?' said Dr Susan.

'It would be good to meet people I used to know and, of course, even more reason for following a moral path beforehand.'

'What about judgement?' said Dr Strait. 'Aren't you afraid of that?'

'There are things I regret,' said Dr Shorts, 'but if God exists, there has to be forgiveness.'

'Definitely,' said Dr Susan.

'So, getting back to the patients: if it's true that self-understanding helps us to relate to the position of others, I think it will help for us all to entertain different standpoints within ourselves. Susan, perhaps you could try and understand agnosticism, as well as other religious faiths.'

'I'm sure every Christian has doubts. That's why we depend on faith, and I've come to believe that there are many possible pathways to God. I'm sure he takes people as they come.'

'And you, Dai, might entertain agnosticism, if only to relate to the patients. You're always being angry with God for all the bad things that happen, but it's illogical to be angry with someone who's not there.'

'Quite right, Mr Spock,' said Dr Strait. 'That seems to have sorted out Mr Choleric and Mr Tidy, if not the rest of humanity!'

'What about Mrs Liszt,' said Dr Susan. 'She seems to be too busy to be worried about death.'

Keeping busy is one way of avoiding uncomfortable thoughts, isn't it? I'm sure you guys all have patients with multiple complaints, many of them investigated up to the hilt. As we've previously discussed, Freud would probably have put them down to sexual hang-ups.

'Have you asked her about her sex life?' said Dr Strait.
'Then she can go on the waiting list for psychosexual counselling,' said Dr Shorts.
'Yet another referral to swell her bulging file!' said Dr Susan.

Multiple symptoms might have different meanings in different individuals, just as non-verbal behaviour can also be ambiguous. Both represent the release of energy. It needn't necessarily be sexual energy. You might be interested to know that Freud, in his later writings, backed away somewhat from the sexual track. At least, he redefined the concept to include almost everything about life. He called it *Eros*, the life force, as opposed to *Thanatos*, disintegration and death.

'Being ready to try and understand her as another person,' said Dr Susan. 'That's what she needs. It's just the same as all the others really. Just like the paintings, too.'
'And not being afraid,' said Dr Shorts.
'So you've answered your own question,' said Dr Strait.

Guys, it's getting late. I think we should go home, but next time I want to look at how the artist provokes responses in other individuals through the language of the paint.

'Not too many bullet points here!' says Donald.
'Wait and see,' says Liam. 'There's a whole chapter later on, just for you!'

References

1   Smith A (1987) Mark Rothko in retrospect. *The Antique Collector*. **July**: 58.

2   Elkins J (2004) *Pictures and Tears*. Routledge, New York and London.

3   Breslin J (1993) *Mark Rothko, a biography*. University of Chicago Press, Chicago.

4   Bronowski J (1977) *The Ascent of Man*. Book Cub Associates, London.

5   Freud S and Breuer J (1976) *Studies in Hysteria*. Penguin, London.

6   Freud S (1976) *The Interpretation of Dreams*. Penguin, London.

7   Sylvester D (1975) *The Brutality of Fact: interviews with Francis Bacon*. Thames and Hudson, London, re-printed 1987.

Resource

Middleton E (1995) *The Art of Suffering* (dissertation). Loughborough University, School of Art and Design. Unpublished.

CHAPTER 7

Paint language

Paint is a metaphorical rather than a literal language. The manner of application, influenced both by conscious and unconscious drivers, gives rise to dynamics that reflect the artist's inner reality. These have the potential of connecting directly, without words, with the inner world of the observer. It may help for non-painters to imagine the body language of the artist as they apply the paint.

'Are there bullet points in this chapter?' says Donald.
'Not many,' says Liam, 'but lots of sludgy marks.'

'I'll grant you that these artists are capable of stirring up thoughts and feelings, as we saw in the last meeting,' said Dr Strait, 'but what I really want to know is how they do it.'
'The language of the paint that our tutor kept mentioning,' said Dr Susan. 'I'd love to learn how to read it.'
'But I don't think that it's like translating from French or German into English,' said Dr Shorts.

Not a bit like that, guys! You must understand that paint is a metaphorical language: it is not so much the subject or story depicted, as *how* it is painted.

'Like jokes,' says Donald. 'It's the way I tell 'em.'
'That's the trouble,' says Liam.

The way paint is applied can be a metaphor for an entire range of emotions, in the most expressive artworks. In certain contexts, a rapidly changing paint surface equates with a range of emotional responses to the imagery. To gauge the paint language, try looking not at each part, so much as at juxtapositions. For example: not the hair, the arm, the dress – but the highlight of the hair in relation to the tone and brush strokes of the background right next to the hair, and how this changes as we move further away from the hair. Scanning from left to right, up and down, plus observing the very edges of a painting can all be informative. This develops an awareness of the potential for paint to communicate in its own right, independently of, and yet in conjunction with, the subject.

Paint language is a combination of conscious and unconscious use of paint. The tension between conscious (e.g. subject, scale of work) and unconscious decisions (e.g. certain sorts of brushwork, echoes of rhythms, ambiguous shapes) gives a certain frisson to the painting: its compelling potential to communicate. It's as if conscious decisions set the scene, from which the unconscious takes its cues. As a painter, it's when you stop thinking as such, that the unconscious input is more likely to come through. In my experience this is more likely to happen several hours into painting, when the cares of everyday life are completely non-existent.

To draw a theatrical parallel, Antonin Artaud[1] thought that, far from furthering human achievement, psychology had caused a fearful loss (of energy) by persisting in bringing the unknown down to a level with the known. He illustrated this by stating that actors no longer knew how to scream, they did nothing but talk. Artaud was all for the affective, rather than illustrative, route of communication, because he wanted to cause a physical response in the observer *first*. Cognition could come later.

'That's like dreams and the unconscious,' said Dr Shorts.
'According to Freud,' said Dr Strait.
'As we agreed at the last meeting,' said Dr Susan.

Let's hear it from Francis Bacon:

'You know, in my case, all painting – and the older I get, the more it becomes so – is an accident. So I foresee it in my mind – I foresee it, and yet I hardly ever carry it out as I foresee it. *It transforms itself by the actual paint* [my italics]. I use very large brushes, and in the way I work I don't in fact know very often what the paint will do, and it does many things which are very much better than I could make it do. Is that an accident? Perhaps one could say it's not an accident, because it becomes a selective process which part of this accident one chooses to preserve'.[2]

So Bacon's paintings can be seen in terms of a balance between chance and order. Bacon again:

'The other day I painted a head of someone . . . the paint moving from one contour into another made a likeness . . . the next day I tried to take it further . . . and I lost the image completely'.[2]

Bacon refers to painting like this as,

'a kind of tightrope walk between what is called figurative painting and abstraction . . . It's an attempt to bring the figurative thing up onto the nervous system more violently and more poignantly'.[2]

This supports Novitz's view[3] that the 'best' art is 'transparent', leading the eager intellect to a direct apprehension of 'reality' – inner reality. In his view the 'worst' art emphasises appearances, and excludes the reality it purports to reveal. The 'best' art becomes 'reality', whilst life itself (the external world) becomes a pale imitation of art.

I think that the most valuable component of painting is that communicated through the unconscious. Otherwise painting would just be straightforward illustration, and I would never have become captivated. The artist's unconscious has the potential to trigger recognition with that of the spectator, through touching deeper levels without words. It's the deeper levels of being alive that matter: beauty and truth. Therefore catalogues in art exhibitions function as a barrier between me and these deeper levels. I do recognise, of course, that catalogues have their place as useful sources of information, but when being 'fed' and nurtured by art via the unconscious, to be diverted through catalogue words usually strikes me as a meagre and often irrelevant translation into an inappropriate language.

'You need to make a connection with the art in some way,' said Dr Susan, 'although catalogues often seem to be heavy going – rather like a history lesson.'

Learning how to get something out of the paint alone is like learning a new language. You could call it simply 'technique', but 'paint language' is more 'speaking', complex and nuanced than simply one technique as opposed to another. Of course it helps if you speak the language too (i.e. are a painter), but as a non-practitioner getting to grips with it: imagine the sort of physical activity required to create the marks which make up the painting. Relate this paint language to body language, matching the physical activity needed to make the marks to an appropriate state of mind. Consider this in relation to the subject and you are getting close to understanding how the painter felt about that subject.

Standing in front of a painting you like in an art gallery, you might trace some marks in the air, in front of the painting, as if you are the artist. Try to get the speed of the brushstrokes right. Imagine the paint consistency and try to become the painter, as it were.

'Sounds like a good way to get locked up!' said Dr Strait.
'I should think the attendants would be worried that you might be going to damage the painting!' said Dr Shorts.
'But I think I've seen people doing that in art galleries,' said Dr Susan. 'They must have been painters.'
'Or pretending to be!' said Dr Strait.

Look for brushstrokes which have been done at speed, and areas where the paint seems to have been applied repeatedly (i.e. layers, which means 'visited' a lot). This doesn't necessarily indicate unconscious communication, since the artist could have been working at speed under time or financial pressures, or it could indicate some problem with underlying drawing or handling of the medium. However, the instinctive handling of an area, fuelled by the unconscious, can't be ruled out.

Consider textural (paint texture) differences and relationships of different elements in the composition – what is juxtaposed with what? Imagine the touch: what is the painter enjoying and, by extension, what is he inviting the patron or spectator to enjoy too? Remember when looking at old art, that modern 'consumers' were not in mind – the patron would be a wealthy high status individual, who commissioned the art, specifying preferences (e.g. subject, pose) and constraints (e.g. financial).

Another tack is to consider painting in terms of energy. To quote John on non-verbal communication: 'I don't know what's going on, but sure as hell, something is'.[4]

'That's Mrs Liszt,' said Dr Susan.
'And do we really want to know what's going on with her?' said Dr Strait.

Find the part of the painting that appears to have been done with the most energy. Chances are, that this is the bit that engaged the painter the most. Also it's likely that some of the marks were applied more quickly than can be done with conscious decision at every move. This, then, is where the unconscious is likely to reside.

Are there any anatomical contours that have been re-worked to increase emphasis? Look at the painting in raking light if possible to identify different thicknesses and layers of paint. Sometimes this is due to redefining a contour, or to *pentimenti* (changes of mind/corrections during the evolution of a painting).

'Temperamental!' says Donald.
'No, pentimenti!' says Liam.
'Petulant and mental,' says Donald. 'It's the same thing!'

But alternatively many layers means a place re-visited many times and is likely to indicate repeated pleasure. Painting is a tactile pursuit and brushstrokes are strokes. Look at the edges of the painting in terms of thickness of paint, compared with the part that seems most 're-visited'.

That painting is a sensual activity is well known. In his book *What Painting Is*,[5] James Elkins entitles one chapter *Coagulating, cohabiting, macerating, reverberating* – and he's only talking about painting!

A few of us painters make our own oil paints from genuine pigments, which takes much longer than squeezing tubes of paint. The pay-off is inspiration – each colour is pure and unadulterated without commercial bulking additives. Each is beautiful and sings its own exquisite song on the palette alone, before you even do anything with it. I always salivate a bit when preparing my palette, which takes about 20 minutes. And that's another thing: notice any physical changes you experience when looking at art; if something happens it means the art is working – and you're getting it directly, without the help of a catalogue, audio guide, information board or label.

'Please can I go home, Miss?' says Donald. 'I think I need a cold shower!'

Into the paint on the palette we dip/push/scrub an assortment of sticks with hair on the end. Other things are also dipped into the wet colour, like rags or fingers. Every mark that is made affects the next mark. What was clear in our mind at the start soon becomes fraught with complications. Should we leave that unintended mark/colour, or knock it out and follow the narrow path? There is a real, dynamic and continual communication going on 'at the coal face' between the artist's intention, and the materials and their 'intention' to be themselves.

During the course of a painting I am working towards some sort of resolution. Generally speaking, the longer each individual session lasts, the deeper the level of engagement – the best work sometimes emerges almost effortlessly, some hours later. Ideally, satisfactory resolution gains momentum towards the end of a painting, when I sense the end is coming. Suddenly I realise I've arrived, and there is nothing more to be done. At the end of a painting session I clean up and return in small stages to everyday life, on a good day emerging tired and satisfied. To further the discussion of paint language we can view *Lady Agnew of Lochnaw* (1892) by John Singer Sargent, which hangs in the Scottish National Gallery, Edinburgh.

> www.natgalscot.ac.uk – online collections – artists A–Z – select 'S' then Sargent.

The Agnews were an established aristocratic family. Their seat, at Lochnaw in Scotland, had been in the family for nearly 600 years. They spent the season in London where Sargent painted this portrait. Perhaps the esteem in which Sir Noel Agnew held his wife is illustrated by the enormous cost incurred to secure a major artist – for his own portrait he used photography, and later on, a minor artist. Sir Noel touchingly kept meticulous records of the progress of his wife's portrait in his diary, and when it was exhibited in the Royal Academy he went to visit it at least six times. From his diaries, it seems that his wife reluctantly agreed to marriage after an earlier refusal. Significantly, non-specific maladies and fatigue plagued her intermittently ever since.

'Mrs Liszt again?' said Dr Susan.
'We should marry her off to Mr Tidy!' said Dr Strait.

But this did not stop her being a great success as a society hostess, and *The Times* (1932) stated that she was 'an excellent conversationalist and enjoyed a good argument' in contrast with her husband's diary reports of his wife's listlessness.

'What can it all mean, doctor?' said Dr Strait.
'No lists?' said Dr Shorts.
'Ho, ho!' said Dr Strait.

Flowers and floral associations suffuse this portrait. Petal-like colours and a predominance of white symbolises the sitter's youth and natural freshness. But, in a

Freudian interpretation, to hold a bloom in the hand symbolises both 'innocence and sexual sinfulness'.[6] Lady Agnew's white flower head (almost overblown) is held at her genitals. She has an enigmatic facial expression. Whilst presenting an irreproachable face to the world, the steadfast gaze and determined mouth take on alternative associations when linked with pictorial components like frills and transparent fabrics. The chair and hanging drapery are Japanese silk, decorated with floral motifs which associate the sitter with the exotic, contributing to the depiction of wealth and erotic sensuousness. *This painting is about the tactile relationships between silks, satins, taffeta, nubile flesh and gold,* rather than a record of who Lady Agnew was. Power is symbolised through possessions and beauty, not by assertive body language, and Lady Agnew's sexual power is all the more potent for being presented in such a languorous way. The hanging arm holds the rhythmic, buttoned chair edge suggestively and she looks straight at you. Blatant sexuality tempered by respectability and decorum.

'Wow!' said Dr Shorts. 'What would you do – faced with a model like that?'
'Not listless, anyway!' said Dr Susan. 'At least, not according to Sargent.'

This portrait supports Andrew Wilton's description of the 'best' modern portraiture as having, 'as strong an emphasis on the character of the artist as on that of the sitter'.[7] This idea had already been expressed more categorically by Oscar Wilde: 'Every portrait that is painted with feeling is a portrait of the artist, not the sitter'.[8] Kilmurray and Ormond state: 'that he [Sargent] was a physical and sensual kind of person is clear from the whole tenor of his work'.[9]

'So it's all in the mind of the artist?' said Dr Shorts.
'I blame Freud for all this!' said Dr Strait.
'Sigmund?' said Dr Susan.
'The whole family!' said Dr Strait.

Sargent's paint language is variable in this portrait. Lady Agnew's face is pivotally placed and highly finished – appropriate for depicting her perfect complexion and mesmerizing gaze. That is captivating enough, but what I'm really interested in is what happens elsewhere. Look at the plethora of bravura brushstrokes done at speed, culminating in the sash and its bow (another phallic symbol). Like a displacement activity, the non-aggressive colour muffles the sheer energy here; the agitated excitement. More subtly, the contour of the thigh beneath the skirt is defined by shadow, and there is a quiet lilac reflected shine defining her buttock. The sash almost functions like a mini skirt over the thigh; the hanging pendant draws attention to the cleavage.

'Mmm,' said Dr Susan, uncrossing her legs.

'I'm feeling apprehensive!' says Donald.
'And I'm feeling chilled,' says Liam.

My painting, *Scramble* (1998, Plates 5, 6 and 7, private collection, Britain) illustrates how unconscious associations can work. I had been given a set of traditional scales for Christmas, and was delighted with the imagery in the reflections of the metal bowl, every time I put something in it. When the eggs went in I was struck by the swirls, which seemed vaguely (and fittingly) redolent of reproductive organs – but that's as far as I consciously thought. I just painted it because the imagery was stimulating.

After the painting was completed, the following observations were made: scramble is what fighter pilots do when they take off; like the race of the sperm to be first at the egg; more generally it is life's struggle (finding a life partner, the career ladder); the whole composition is reminiscent of a surgical table, with metal receptacle and knife; there is a dynamic energy (because it's a bit awkward and top-heavy) from bottom to top; the bowl points upwards, the knife, wood grain and overall format are vertical and the high viewpoint accentuates this; the bowl is a scrotum with testes; reflections are vasa deferentia; the egg box is an ovary, the two empty spaces representing discharged eggs. The unconscious is multi-layered and ambiguous, so don't expect things to add up logically.

'Wait a minute!' said Dr Strait, 'Some people read anything into art. It's only a still life.'
'Perhaps the artist should have the last say,' said Dr Susan.

Well as far as I'm concerned you can drop the fighter pilots and life's struggle, but the rest I think probably was working its way into the painting, filtering up through the unconscious.

A new student will typically turn up at one of my painting classes to learn the 'proper techniques' for oil painting. In order to start at where the learner is I comply and introductory exercises are undertaken. However, as soon as possible I explain that intention is everything, and that this is what determines so-called 'technique'. To contemplate your relationship to your subject is the best start: what is it you want to say through painting? Some build-up of frustrated energy is useful, because fired up sufficiently, everything else will follow. All techniques were, of course, once experiments – by artists whose expressive need wasn't catered for by existing media or methods. The invention of oil paint, in contrast with the older egg tempera, for example, enabled the artist to blend colours with incomparable smoothness, luminosity and lusciousness over several hours. By contrast, egg tempera dries quickly, making later alterations noticeable.

Whilst some paint language is arrived at unconsciously, there is always a 'business' side to making paintings, in terms of deciding which materials to use. Even before we think about the colour and tonal overall scheme, scale, support (e.g. canvas? wood panel?) and type of surface will need to be considered. There are a great variety of paint surfaces available commercially, but I make my own – each panel receives eight layers of gesso (an ancient mixture of whiting and titanium white, bound in warm rabbit skin glue). The reason I go to such lengths is that gesso is a beautiful surface to work on, having just the right degree of porosity, allowing for great luminosity to stream through glaze layers, and being tough enough to tolerate plenty of rubbing through to the gesso itself for highlights. Luminosity comes from the depths of a painting.

At every turn decisions have to be made. The complexity of this experience can only really be appreciated by a practising artist. It can drive you mad, too, because what you first had in mind is so elusive, because new and tempting paths open up instead (shall I take that unexpected new and rather exciting route, or knock it out and stay on the straight and narrow?), and because the unconscious also has its own ideas. In short, it is a heady mix, but the point is that paint language is both consciously and unconsciously arrived at. There is a constant tension which Duchamp, talking about art in general, described as being 'like an arithmetical relation between the unexpressed but intended, and the unintentionally expressed'.[10]

'Poor rabbits!' said Dr Susan.
'But don't you think it's a kind of immortality?' said Dr Shorts
'What? – ending up as a layer of gesso?'
'Yes, but in a great painting!'
'You're both mad!' said Dr Strait.

Tree of Life II (Plate 8) was made as a development from, and in response to, the weaknesses of *Tree of Life I* (Plate 2, *see* Chapter 4). I desired a large allegorical portrait of our family, with energy rather than stasis. It combines straightforward imagery, symbolism and paint language. The weaknesses, this time, are some poorly observed underlying drawing and too much high colour contrast, which means that each colour is not able to sing its song, for being drowned out by the others. For the next in this series, I may add more neutrals, to counterbalance the high chroma hues, and I need to do more preliminary studies with closer direct observation of the subjects.

'I like the bright colours,' said Dr Susan.
'A bit psychedelic for me, I'm afraid,' said Dr Strait.

In this painting, which stands 171cm tall, each member of the nuclear family appears twice. The arch format immediately puts it into a quasi classical-religious mode. The central self-portrait (Plate 9), my head emerging from a tree trunk, is the matriarchal pivotal point. The painting was begun before, and finished a few months after, my total ankle replacement. Of all my operations this was the most enduringly painful, and it shows in the face. The deformed foot is exposed as the stallion performs the *lavade*, under which, in tiny writing, is the operation date. Frida Kahlo used to write words on her paintings in a similar way. The Lady Godiva imagery accosts John as he receives inspiration (based on Rodin's *The Age of Bronze*).

John contemplates and creates, as a musical parallel to Bellori's (Italian art historian 1615–96) concept of *The Idea* (Plate 10).[11] Bellori's belief, writing about visual art, was that perfect beauty does not exist in nature and must be sought instead in the realm of Ideas, whereby intellect is 'animated by imagination'.[12]

John is surrounded by his score, the *St. John Passion*, some notes and words of which are faithfully detailed. Beneath this is everyday John, playing one of his guitars, and beneath him, our vet student daughter. Bottom right is the Broadwood baby grand piano, now over 100 years old, inherited from my grandmother who received it as a wedding present and used to teach on it. Above its lid, stand Anthony and Rachael as toddlers, on our landing stage on the river, at the bottom of our garden. Above that is Anthony as performer, wearing a mask bought in Venice. He is in a shaft of light, reminiscent of stage lighting.

The tree has become a series of expressive lines, and here is a route from narrative to more 'psychological' ways of understanding. The great central trunk is made up of countless glazes (thin translucent veils of colour) to build up a rich colour resonance and image of strength, reminiscent of those great western American 600 year old red cedars. The arabesque boughs lend a lyricism to the imagery contained within. Distant branches become slightly tortured, reaching out, grasping, a bit desperate. So the rich fabric of family life which we all share on some level, can be 'read' through the nature of the tree components alone. The pastoral river scene is contrasted opposite my head with an undefined red area. This didn't really come off, but was meant to work both as a contrast to graphic imagery, such as the musical score, whilst also representing the opposite of gentle pastoral – the negative energy of anxiety.

'Artists are very self-critical, aren't they?' said Dr Shorts.
'Some of them not enough so!' said Dr Strait.
'Don't be such a misery!' said Dr Susan.

Areas of hair also begin to express themselves through the paint as well as the imagery, i.e. *how* an area is painted becomes as important as *what* is painted. After all, if the only point is to produce a straightforward image, why paint at all? These days, what can paint do that digital imagery can't? Is there anything left? Why yes, the mark of the painter, the texture, the 'hand on it' factor. In *Tree of Life II*, there is energy in my stallion's mane as it's built up with relative speed by *scumbling* (dry-ish paint applied on top of rough dry paint, catching the tops only of the previous hard layer of paint). It rushes down, gushing over my leg. Conversely, the girl rider's hair symbolises innocence, being a broad white-ish brushstroke. My hair become clean sweeps of flat intensified colour, symbolising energy – in painting you can do anything, become anyone, it's a form of freedom.

'Escapism!' says Donald.
'From what?' says Liam.
'Reality,' says Donald.
'Ah, but what is reality?' says Liam.

I will conclude my own work by looking at paintings that incorporate the ancient craft of *gilding*. The imagery within the 2005 series of about 20 gilded paintings sometimes appears lighter, sometimes darker, than the gold or silver leaf. The paint is made from genuine pigments bound in oil, in small volumes made for the day's painting only. Genuine pigments, especially transparent ones, give a degree of clarity that tube paint usually doesn't because of various 'pollutant' additives designed to extend the shelf life up to 10 years.

Conceptually these paintings function on a number of levels, held in balance.

Our Daily Bread *(2005) (Plate 1, private collection, Britain)*

- Wholesome food; domesticity – traditional values.
- Visually engaging – relationships between thick bread textures, gold leaf and the sharp clarity of the knife. Colour values (warm bread; cool knife).
- Christian connections: title and Byzantine icon associations. Celebrating the everyday, raising its status.
- Sexual – the 'female' bread; the 'male' knife.
- Distressed gold leaf has a different expressiveness to faultless gilding: the 'lived in' feel, like a kindly mature face.

Fish for Dinner *(2005) (Plate 11, private collection, United Arab Emirates)*

- Silver plated cutlery painted to look more silver than the silver leaf it's on. Tonal challenges: the iridescence of fish scales in relation to highlights elsewhere, holding the thing in light/dark balance: a study in the nature of silver.
- Christian associations: the fish as reminiscent of the feeding of the 5000 (a recurring theme). The upwards emphasis is commonly used in western religious painting.
- Surreal – in everyday life the fish would be on a plate, not suspended in spatial ambiguity. To remove objects from their usual setting can encourage us to look at them afresh. Discover the extraordinary in the ordinary.

'It's all a bit religious,' said Dr Strait.
'What about the Freudian stuff?' said Dr Shorts.
'I don't think all upright images are phallic symbols,' said Dr Susan, 'whatever Freud may say.'

Knife Trio *(2005) (Plate 12, collection of the artist)*

- Crucifixion associations.
- Associations with domestic violence. Also when viewed, your own vague reflection appears behind the vertical knives, ensnaring you – my own head shape can be made out as I took the photograph.

- Tonal study – the lack of high intensity hues draws attention to subtle tonal nuances of gold in relation to earth colours.
- The simple beauty of domestic objects: handles you want to hold.

'I've always been scared of kitchens!' says Donald.
'In case you were asked to wash up!' says Liam.

Finally, I would like to have a brief look at the work of some of the 'old masters', in relation to their paint language. The following paintings are in the National Gallery, London.

Decent quality large images can be attained via www.nationalgallery.org.uk
Go to: Collections – Full Collection Index – Select first letter of artist's surname – click on 'image', and again to enlarge it.

Peter Paul Rubens: Samson and Delilah *(c.1609)*

This painting was commissioned to hang in the 'Great Saloon' of Nicolaas Rockox who was the burgomaster of Antwerp.

The story: Delilah is offered 1100 pieces of silver by the Philistines to discover the secret of Samson's superhuman strength, which would lead to their capture of him. She seduces him, which results in his confiding to her that his strength lies in his hair – if it's cut off he will lose his strength. Delilah betrays him, and the barber cuts off Samson's hair as he slumbers, exhausted with love-making. Through the door, we see the Philistines in the distance, waiting to capture Samson.

The scene that Rubens paints is highly charged, and the paint language contributes to this: we get the meaning twice: through imagery and through the qualities of the paint itself. The hot overall colour scheme sets the general atmosphere at once. The lusciousness of the foreground red and gold draperies speak loud and clear of emotional sensuality, their very folds functioning as metaphorical depths of warmth and luxury. It's the *way* it's painted, at full throttle as it were, with a brush loaded with rich pigment bound in glossy oil. The smoothing and caressing of it during the act of painting must have been deeply enjoyed by Rubens – you can't paint like that in a detached sort of way. The bare flesh and hair of Delilah are studies in erotic delight. Golden ringlets trickle over a perfect complexion. The palpable breasts are stressed by the clothing surrounding them. Her prominent shoulder almost functions as another breast because of the way the light describes the form. Samson's flesh is browner than hers, to emphasize her white nudity, his massive hanging arm a metaphor in itself, I suspect. Against this overt heat and slumbering lusciousness, the aggressive glint of the alert Philistines' armour gives a sharp clash – it didn't have to, this area could have been painted slightly out of focus.

How on earth did the Puritan burgomaster of the city get away with hanging such an emotive image in such a conspicuous position within his home, which would have been frequented by the good and the great? Ah yes, because the painter and patron were relying on the mindsets of other Puritans, who observed the painting, not owning to dwelling on the subliminal, but taking the Old Testament story (Judges 16:4–20) at face value.

'Honi soit qui mal y pense!' said Dr Strait.
'I didn't know you were a Latin scholar,' said Dr Shorts.

Peter Paul Rubens: Portrait of Susanna Lunden *(c.1622–5)*

Rubens' ideal *femme fatale* shares some similarities with this portrait of his future sister-in-law. One can only wonder what his fiancé made of it. Rubens seems to have had a thing about stressed breasts – this time they are pushed just beneath her chin, off-set with luscious red fabric. Their pearlescent quality is achieved through carefully orchestrated lighting, and the succession of thin translucent veils of oily paint called *glazes*. Each layer contributes to the complex and subtle nuances. In other words Rubens would have 're-visited' this area probably more than any other in this painting. Look at the contrast between the way the breasts are handled, and the hands, for example. Paint language can be revelatory about a painter's sexuality, not simply because of what is depicted, but the qualities.

Paul Delaroche: The Execution of Lady Jane Grey *(1833)*

Lady Jane Grey was the great-granddaughter of Henry VII. Following the death of Edward VI in 1553 she reigned as queen for nine days before being disposed of by the supporters of Mary Tudor, tried for treason and beheaded at Tower Hill in 1554 (*see* Chapter 4).

Here it's the paint language of Lady Jane's dress that is doing the talking. The white satin works on a number of levels. White traditionally denotes innocence, including virginity. It's the first thing that hits you in this painting, because of the huge tonal contrast between it and everything else. The successive glazes, which describe the sensuous and complex folds, are built up to such a degree that it is as if the dress is crying out for you to touch it. Furthermore, the body beneath the fabric is easy to discern. Her blindfold contributes to the blatant sexuality of this image, as does the long golden hair falling over one shoulder, giving her a slightly wanton look. Yes, of course she is about to be beheaded but, on a subliminal level, is the virgin being 'offered' to the Paris Salon visitor? If you think that's going a bit far, why isn't she in a much less exotic dress of a darker colour? That alone would calm the image down whilst the narrative would remain unaltered.

'Another excuse for men to ogle women!' said Dr Susan.
'Like 'Pan's People',' said Dr Strait.
'Pan's who?' said Dr Shorts.

Rembrandt van Rijn: Belshazzar's Feast *(1636–8)*

Another piece of clothing here: Belshazzar's mantle. It didn't have to be painted in an impasto (very thick) turmoil of painterly excitement, in fact it could have been done using the same method as Lady Jane Greys' dress. But Rembrandt wanted a different sort of excitement – that of panic.

The subject comes from chapter five of the Old Testament Book of Daniel. At a feast, the idolatrous King of Babylon uses precious utensils looted from the Temple of God at Jerusalem. Suddenly the hand of God appears, writing the fatal words in Hebrew which translated mean: 'You have been weighed in the balance and found to be wanting', referring to Belshazzar's imminent death. At this, the Old Testament tells us: 'the king's countenance was changed ... and his knees smote one against the other'. As Neil MacGregor argues – Rembrandt uses the very surface of the paint to describe panic: 'It is as if the paint itself were over-wrought, tormented and distressed ... if we look more closely at the gold encrus-tations of the king's cloak, they become themselves a metaphor of violence.'[12] MacGregor goes on to describe in some detail how this unique surface was arrived at – a series of identifiable stages are passed through, culminating in 'the unin-hibited climax to a long and controlled workshop process.' There would seem to be a tension here, between control and 'let rip', as MacGregor puts it. Paint lan-guage at its highest level of communication involves planning as well as instinct.

'I've never really looked at how the paint was applied before,' said Dr Shorts, 'although I guess I was aware of some of it.'
'It's obvious now, that painters must enjoy handling and playing with paint,' said Dr Susan. 'It's the same thing as musicians savouring the qualities of sound.'
'Or poets playing with words.'
'I'm not sure I like all this sexual business underneath it,' said Dr Strait.
'What do you think your patients do when they get home, Dai?' said Dr Shorts.
'Do I need to know?' said Dr Strait.

'It's nothing but voyeurism!' says Donald.
'A question of degree, surely?' says Liam.
'What does that mean?'

'Just that doctors, at least GPs, have to engage with their patients' lives in order to understand them. How much is a matter of judgement, of course, but the arts can help give a sense of perspective – and maybe an outlet.'
'Speak for yourself!' says Donald.

Well guys, we have come to the end of our practical sessions on paintings and their meanings. It remains to try and tie up what you have learned with applications to professional development and teaching (*see* section on general visual analysis in Chapter 8.)

References

1   Artaud A (1970) *The Theatre and its Double*. Calders and Boyars, London.

2   Sylvester interview with Francis Bacon. In: Harrison C and Wood P (1996) *Art in Theory 1900 – 1990: an anthology of changing ideas*. Blackwell, London.

3   Novitz D (1990) Art, life and reality. *British Journal of Aesthetics*. 30(4): 301.

4   Middleton J. (2000) *The Team Guide to Communication*. Radcliffe Medical Press, Oxford.

5   Elkins J (1999) *What Painting is*. Routledge, New York and London.

6   Freud S (1977) *The Interpretation of Dreams*. Penguin, London (original publication 1900).

7   Wilton A (1992) *The Swagger Portrait*. Tate Gallery, London.

8   Wilde O (1891) *The Picture of Dorian Gray*. London: Richter; 1891. Chapter 1.

9   Kilmurray E and Ormond R (1998) *John Singer Sargent*. Tate Gallery, London.

10 Duchamp M (1957) *The Creative Act*. The Convention of the American Federation of Arts, Texas.

11 Fernie E (1998) *Art History and its Methods*. Phaidon Press, London. From Giovanni Bellori's *Lives of the Modern Painters, Sculptors and Architects* of 1672 (original text).

12 MacGregor N (1997) *Making Masterpieces*. BBC and The National Gallery, London.

Resources

- Erica Middleton's website www.minigallery.co.uk/Erica_Middleton

- Middleton E (2000) *Artistic Integrity and Patronage in Two Portraits by John Singer Sargent* (MA dissertation). University of Nottingham. Unpublished.

CHAPTER 8

Paintings and personal professional development

Concentrate on the art that nourishes you. First let the painting 'speak' to your emotions. Give it enough time. Your reactions are as valid as those of anyone else. Analyse the 'meanings', or read the guide book later. Reflections on art can be incorporated into a log, informing your personal learning plan.

Personal development

Choosing how you are going to develop means looking at how you are currently presenting yourself, who you really are and who you would like to become. The journey through life can facilitate some developments whilst marginalising previous characteristics. The roles that we fulfil in middle age are probably very different to those from our youth, and we have almost certainly had to reinvent ourselves over and over again. Some of us, especially approaching old age, may feel that self-understanding is more about who we are spiritually, rising above material and physical concerns. Whatever our 'take' on this subject, uninvited life and perception-changing events happen to us all sooner or later.

Some of us, perhaps more so women, may be able to increase self-awareness through absorbing an artist such as Kahlo (*see* Chapter 5). Just give it enough time – some art can have a quiet, haunting power. Kahlo may enable some of us to recognise understated parts of ourselves, nurturing and drawing us along, and by extension we may be better equipped to recognise and empathise with the crises of others.

For me, this is the enduring pull of art; it has the power to nourish through exposure to great beauty, through great perception, through extending and developing my understanding of who I am, and who I am becoming, with the passing of time. Art replenishes emotional fatigue. I like to think this all helps me to reach out to others in their plight, and that I might be of more use to them than I would have been without art, which opened my eyes to deeper nuances of human experience. But actually it's more selfish than that – art which stops me in my tracks is the thing, to be spoken to piercingly and unerringly, and sometimes when you're least expecting it. Here, I am speaking as an artist, not as a health professional.

However, there's another route too, the haunting influence, much quieter than the lightening bolt. Works of art can reveal themselves slowly, really slowly, over years and even decades, exposing different nuances of themselves as we ourselves change (as an artist, as well as a person). They become old friends, saying different things to me at different stages of my life, always there to be emotionally lent on – reassurance, continuity. 'Hi there again, beautiful painting. Glad you're still around.'

How to look at an exhibition of paintings

In order to get the most out of an exhibition, my belief is that you need to focus on that which really nourishes you and only scan the rest. Imagine being given a snippet of music, a few seconds of a play/film, a few words from a novel – then onto another snippet. Other art forms don't compete in the way that paintings hanging in an exhibition do. Consider how long the painter might have taken to create a given painting. Observe how long people tend to stand in front of a painting within an art gallery – huge discrepancy. At least with music, plays, films or books you are a captive audience for a while and therefore by definition you give time. Give a painting enough time!

My motivation to visit a temporary exhibition is always as a painter. What I'm really after is that which has the potential to develop and extend me as an artist. I love visual beauty – this is what brought me to art in the first place as a child and has remained my overriding motivation ever since. Passing through the exhibition I don't think in words, but get drawn and immersed instead. Words come later, when sharing experience with others.

I can only take in so much at a time at this intense level, and the trick is to reach your destination 'blind' – behold what you came for before you are fatigued by everything else. That way you get the unique input at full throttle. It stays with you – in my case for years. That's the fuel and the nourishment I seek. Nothing else is as valuable.

As medics you may like to parallel this. What is it that really speaks to you? What draws you along and develops you as a person? Here's how to maximise the input. It's the way I've been visiting temporary exhibitions for decades now. I have in mind large-scale temporary London exhibitions – permanent collections can be accessed repeatedly and so attention can be given to different works on different occasions.

1   Go alone. It's all too easy to treat visiting an art gallery as a social event, but if you go with anyone else your experience will be compromised. It's between you and the artist.

2   Don't hire an audio guide: it will wreck the potential of being transported. If you buy a guide book/catalogue don't look at it in front of the art. Written meanings dilute visual experience, and usually they are constructed by someone other than the artist. Artists express themselves in another language, so don't allow an alien one to interfere. Over a coffee later could be the time to absorb post-modern, contextual meanings. But remember: what they say is as valid as what you think – you too are a professional, and the most interesting contemporary art history often comes from other walks of life than from 'pure' art historians. The meaning of art is negotiable, depending on who engages with it: you too have an important role in determining meaning. This is why it's the eyes and the mind which matter, and nothing should be allowed to get in the way.

3   Don't start at the beginning of the exhibition. Usually there's a crowd in front of the first painting, with audio guides, pamphlets and jostling. That prevents quiet contemplation, which, in fact may be impossible to achieve anywhere in a major temporary exhibition. Walk through each room quite briskly, scanning the walls, noting what is where, but at the same time *do* allow yourself to be deflected from your mission by the beautiful, the astonishing, the outrageous. The paintings which speak most eloquently are likely to be towards the end of the exhibition, as they are usually organised chronologically, ending with a great climax in the famous works. So it's a sort of race to get where you need to be without being 'hijacked' on the way.

So here you are, in front of what you came for, still fresh to absorb. A really good exhibition might have just three or four paintings which really speak to you. In front of these, don't think at all, just bathe in the imagery. What was it that made the painter want to paint this? (Do you love it too?) Where is the most energy, the most excitement? The most paint layers? The most expressively articulated? The most beautiful juxtapositions and relationships?

Consider these relationships – not only human relationships depicted, but passages across different parts of the whole. Has the painter revealed something to you? Commit imagery to memory – to call on in the future, the way the artist (and you) felt when confronted by this sort of flesh/this kind of interior/this colour or lighting. One of my painting tutors has become a close friend. When we come across striking imagery we often communicate our appreciation via an artist's name/period only – to say 'early van Gogh' is enough: he has taught us how to love and respect the rough hands, the weathered face in a way less possible before seeing his work.

Relate a painting, which speaks to you, to others in the exhibition – what are the common factors? It might be imagery such as a certain type of figure, or it might be a colour, a certain sort of lighting or a repeated place depicted. In a word, become the painter, feel as he does, know what turns him on. Move with the painter as you trace the main compositional rhythms and localised mark-making of the paint language. Feel first, think later. Experience the nature of paint in its raw state, as a child might – directly, clearly.

Remember John Betjeman:

> 'Childhood is measured out
> By sounds and smells and sights
> Before the dark hour of reason grows.'
> from *Summoned by Bells*

Laura Mulvey,[1] an early feminist, linked types of looking and associated pleasures to gender difference. She cited Freud's *Three Essays on Sexuality*[2] in which he isolated scopophilia as a sexual instinct in which other people are treated like objects, subjecting them to a curious and controlling gaze. Traditionally in painting the man is the spectator, the woman is there to be contemplated: her role is to hold the look, both playing to and signifying male desire. In Frida Kahlo's close-up self portraits (*see* Chapter 5) she simultaneously presents herself as both exotic and sexually desirable whilst being confrontational, thus refusing the designated traditional female role. She's in charge, and not only contemporaneously, but for the future too, for to produce calculated self-imagery is to make a bid for posthumous reputation too. For me, these direct head and shoulder self-portraits speak far more eloquently than the slightly comic-strip flavour of her more graphic narrative imagery regarding subjects such as surgery and abortions.

General visual analysis

The purpose of visual analysis is to take the time to understand an artwork more fully than casual observations allow. There are two components: content and formal elements.

Content is what a painting depicts – what's happening plus the nature/style of the imagery. For example, how are the figures depicted – idealised or naturalistic?

Formal elements are 'the tools of the trade'. By analysing how the artist has used these we can enhance our understanding of the content. Formal elements include: composition, lighting, colour, viewpoint and perspective, painting technique.

As well as the depicted humanity, the other 'humanity' is the response which comes from the artist and is responded to by the viewer. Formal elements are used in very specific ways to facilitate our perception of the artist's standpoint. In this way the artist could be understood in terms of a 'fellow professional'.

Composition

Composition is the main structure of a painting. Are you led through the painting via big rhythms, lines, gestures, repeated colours? What shape do the main compositional lines give? Are these stable (e.g. geometric, symmetrical) or unstable (e.g. diagonal, zig-zag)? Does this contribute to the mood of the content?

Is there a focal point? (a part to which your eye is directed). Why is that bit so important? Are there any subsidiary compositions (like sub-plots) within the main composition?

Lighting

Why light it this way? Consider alternatives, e.g. light from another direction, at another time of day, soft lighting instead of hard, or vice versa.

Where is the maximum tonal (i.e. light/dark) contrast? What effect does this give to the painting as a whole?

Does the lighting/tonal pattern help to accentuate any focal point?

Are all the figures lit the same way? If not, what does this mean?

Colour

What is the colour range – which colours are repeated, which omitted? Consider the relationship of high-low saturation/intensity colours: does this attract our attention to some parts of the painting? Do repeating colours guide the eye round the painting? Might some colours hold symbolic significance?

Viewpoint and perspective

Viewpoint: How near/far are we from the action? How would this feel if we were really in the painting? Do we look straight across or up/down? Does any person hold eye contact with us, and what does this mean?

Perspective: To what extent is the illusion of distance depicted? Is this done through aerial or linear perspective? What effect does this produce in the painting as a whole?

Painting technique

Does the way in which the paint has been applied contribute to our understanding of the imagery? For example, meticulously crafted detail gives a different approach to the imagery than a loose Impressionist rendering. Is the paint evenly applied throughout? Can you see any evidence of re-workings/revisions? (Stand so that the light reflects off the paint surface, and look at contours of heads, limbs for evidence of thicker paint). What was the painter after, in these re-workings?

Feminist visual analysis

The purpose of a feminist visual analysis is to draw attention to the contrasting ways in which the genders have been depicted, with a view to exposing the traditional exploitation of women. In many older paintings containing numbers of figures the contrast is very marked. This would be seen as evidence by feminist art historians of 'the objectification of women' by an implicit male audience, i.e. depicting women as objects of decoration and sexual desire, eliminating their personalities. The plot thickens, of course, when homo-eroticism comes into the equation.

1 Are there any specifically feminine or masculine gestures, poses and facial expressions?
2 What is the environment? Is this significant in terms of gender difference – i.e. is it a female environment, a male one or neutral? How does this impact on the inhabitants?
3 Is the paint language different in the depiction of each gender?
4 Consider this painting in relation to 'the gaze'. Who is looking at who, and where are we (e.g. voyeur 'invited in' by a figure within the painting)?

What sort of person (patron?) do you think this painting is directed at?
   Some of the general visual analysis points can be informative in terms of feminist visual analysis too.

A personal reflective log (Table 8.1)

This is adapted from a log that I use for reflection on clinical issues[3] and could be combined with it. The number of columns can be changed according to personal taste, and the document is ideal for running in the background during consulting sessions. For the arts experiences to be included, you would need either a manual or an electronic notebook that could be taken with you, but the principles are similar.
   As part of my Personal Learning Plan (PLP), I will endeavour to capture more reflections on arts experiences and relate them to clinical practice.

'This is a good way of recording experiences that you might otherwise forget,' said Dr Strait. 'I would find it useful for clinical material as well, but I'm ashamed to admit that I don't know how to set up such a thing on the computer' (see Middleton[3]).
'I like it, too,' said Dr Susan. 'But, then I have always tried to relate to my patients as people.'
'It can be overdone, I think,' said Dr Strait. 'In an ideal world, we would have all the time we needed to do a good clinical job and the people bit as well.'
'But we have seen how patients need more than clinical management. Those cases we discussed illustrate it perfectly,' said Dr Susan. 'The trouble is that,

when I get too interested in the human issues, I soon get miles behind and I'm sure that affects the care of patients who come later.'

'You'll just have to go back to clinical mode when you're running so late,' said Dr Strait.

'Surely it's a matter of judgement, like everything else we do,' said Dr Shorts. 'You have to be self-aware, as we have been discussing. Also, as a professional, you have to keep thinking of the patient's interests – you are in a consulting situation, not an art gallery! That means you have to be able to switch appropriately between clinical and human modes, if I can put it that way.'

'That's not an easy thing to do,' said Dr Susan.

'No, you're right. It's one reason why consulting can be so exhausting, and why we might need the arts to replenish us.'

'So, more self-awareness and judgement,' said Dr Susan.

'Yes, you just have to keep asking yourself – why am I doing this, and for whose benefit?'

'Sometimes you really do have to spend a lot of time, though,' said Dr Susan.

'You're right,' said Dr Strait, 'but if it's every other patient, you're getting the balance wrong.'

'It's a very difficult balance,' said Dr Shorts, 'but I am afraid that the job has become more and more like a production line, and that makes it more difficult for us to relate to people in the way that they often need.'

'We have to hope that the pendulum will swing back the other way,' said Dr Susan. 'In the meantime, I'm very grateful for the guidance we've had on how to use paintings for increased insight and replenishment.'

'Hear, hear!' said Drs. Strait and Shorts.

Table 8.1

Chapter	Artwork	Reflection	Action
4	Paintings by Robert Pope	Patient-centred method: the whole person; patient's illness experience	Use Arts experiences for insights into people
4	*The Execution of Lady Jane Grey* by Paul Delaroche	Victims and family history. The male gaze. Doctors as double agents.	Consider role in relation to gender, family and society
4, 7	*Belshazzar's Feast* by Rembrandt van Rijn	Acceptability of health promotion. Painting panic – control v anarchy.	Write the patient's story: how do they perceive scare stories?
4, 7	*Samson and Delilah* by Peter Paul Rubens	Psychosexual issues. Energy, sensuality and repression	Attend to non-verbal cues

Table 8.1 Continued.

Chapter	Artwork	Reflection	Action
4	*Tree of Life I* by Erica Middleton	Narrative and life events	Respect personal beliefs and values
5	*The Broken Column* by Frida Kahlo	Personal triumph over physical adversity by reinventing the self	Consider this approach to ageing and disability
5	*Scream: a homage to Edvard Munch and all my dead children* by Tracey Emin	Art appealing directly to the emotions. Depression is common in artists and doctors. Performance art cf. Munchausen's syndrome	Consider the patient's illness experience in depression
5	Paintings by Vincent van Gogh	Effects of illness (especially mental illness) on art: would treatment affect creativity?	Reconsider definitions of normality
5, 6, 7	Paintings by Francis Bacon	Legacy of childhood abuse. Sado-masochism and sexual orientation.	Consider the fundamental issue of trust v mistrust
5	*Large Interior, Paddington* by Lucien Freud	Recognition and the meaning of life. Issues of consent.	Consider life scripts in different families and cultures. Re-examine issues of informed consent and use of chaperones
5	*Portrait of Madame X* by John Singer Sargent	Rejection, failure and resilience. Commercial pressures and individual integrity.	Re-examine attitudes to imposed change, threats and opportunities
5	Late self-portraits by Rembrandt van Rijn	Bereavement and loss. Facing death. Pride, stubbornness and political naivety.	Empathy with the unhappy elderly. Take heart from the strength of the human spirit in adversity.
5	Paintings of Peter Paul Rubens	Hard work and political influence leading to success and artistic freedom	Remember to combine the hard work with diplomacy

Table 8.1 Continued.

Chapter	Artwork	Reflection	Action
1, 5, 6	The Seagram Murals by Mark Rothko	Ambiguity and belief. Depression and suicide.	Remember the different faces of depression. Tell patients that they will recover.
7	*Lady Agnew of Lochnaw* by John Singer Sargent	Marital tensions and sexuality: multiple symptoms and malaise	Think of this area when faced with a patient exhibiting similar behaviour
7	*Scramble, Tree of Life II,* Gilded paintings by Erica Middleton	Symbolism, conscious and unconscious dynamics	Remember that artists, doctors and patients are 'wired up' in individual ways
7	*Portrait of Susanna Lunden* by Peter Paul Rubens	Artists revisit favourite areas of the image	Patients' preoccupations are important for them

References

1 Mulvey L (1989) Visual pleasure and narrative cinema. In: *Visual and Other Pleasures.* Macmillan, London (first published 1975).

2 Freud S (1977) *On Sexuality (Three Essays on the Theory of Sexuality).* Penguin, London.

3 Middleton J (2005) A reflective log linked to personal development plans (PDPs) and the practice professional development plan (PPDP). *Education for Primary Care.* **16**: 593–6.

CHAPTER 9

Teaching use of the arts in professional practice

Start from the learner's agenda and recognise that people are 'wired' individually. Arts are not compulsory but people are. Experience of and insight into life is useful for doctors and other health professionals. Difficult cases may generate interest in non-medical approaches. Teachers should begin with art that interests learners, before attempting to stretch them. The aim should be to facilitate the use of an integrated self for the benefit of patients. Working with groups may necessitate compromise, but should not ignore individual expression. Narrative is a useful bridge from medicine to arts, and usually precedes appreciation of paint language and meaning. Recognise and be recognised as fellow travellers: artists, doctors and patients. A curriculum for an 'Arts and Medicine' module is proposed.

Many faces, but one truth

This book is about painting, but similar principles apply across the arts. Let's start with the *face model*: In Chapter 2, I explained how the patient's agenda is important in medical consultations.[1] Well, the model applies equally to the communication in teaching and learning – the agendas are those of the learner and teacher, instead of patient and doctor. Indeed the word 'doctor' also means teacher in relation to health matters.

First principle of education: connect with the learner

That means we must start from where the learner is. So where are they? Who are they? Where do they come from? What do they want? And what do they expect from us? What is the *learner's agenda*?

Not everyone relates to the arts, though many doctors do. Arts is not compulsory, though it may be desirable. There is no point in trying to force it down the throats of the unwilling.

'Are you listening?' says Donald.
'No,' says Liam. 'Anyway, nobody is trying to force you.'

People are not optional though, especially for doctors. How do you understand students with pink spiky hair? Or patients whose problems are about life? *When the learner is ready, the lesson appears*, as Roger Neighbour reminds us.[2]

Learners with a pre-existing interest in the arts may be very ready to make connections with their clinical work, but others will, perhaps, be motivated by a few 'difficult' cases that challenge their assumptions about life.

'Like Mr Tidy,' said Dr Shorts.
'Or Mr Choleric,' said Dr Strait.
'Or Mrs Liszt (*see* Chapter 2). But if we can't find much guidance in our medical
    training, we have to look elsewhere,' said Dr Susan.

Nevertheless, we must recognise that doctors, as well as patients, are 'wired up' in different ways. Not only is there a divide between concrete and imaginative thinkers, but it is quite common for people to relate to some arts and not others. This is reflected in the Myers-Briggs classification of personality types, and in *neurolinguistic programming* – different people appear to be predominantly tuned to visual, physical or sound stimuli.[3,4] For example, musicians don't always like paintings and painters may not care for music. Even an interest in painting rarely means all painting: enthusiasts for the narrative or figurative may find abstract paintings difficult to comprehend.

'Which sort of thinker would you say you are?' says Liam.
'I have a pair of concrete shoes, just your size!' says Donald.

This is not to say that positions are fixed irrevocably. Given the right stimuli and opportunities, many learners can adapt their styles to take in new insights. However, we must value diversity in the learners as well as in the arts. We should try to match the arts experiences with the learners' standpoints.

'You still listening?' says Donald. 'Me and Rothko? I don't think so!'
'Don't forget the goalposts,' says Liam.
'You keep moving them!' says Donald.

If the learner prefers impressionist landscapes to abstract expressionism, we may have to go with that – in order to connect with them. On the other hand, Monet's later paintings begin to resemble abstracts, especially if we take parts of them.

Connecting work and leisure

We may act out different roles at work and off-duty, but these are manifestations of the same self. Our experiences of life are a useful resource for us at work. Using the arts can help to make the connection between life and professional practice stronger. Despite this, some doctors, who are already involved in arts activities, find it difficult to see the relevance to their work. I have noticed this particularly in people who play musical instruments, often to a high standard. What I don't know is whether their expertise is predominantly technical rather than expressive, but it seems to be yet another example of different 'wiring'.

'Scoring goals is a form of self-expression, too,' says Liam.
'You don't fool me,' says Donald. 'I know you're dying to get me back to Tate Modern!'

Multiple and individual agendas

Working with groups of learners is a challenge because their personalities and interests are often diverse. One way of finding out is to start the session by asking individuals to say a little about themselves and their expectations. Sometimes it is possible to achieve a compromise, perhaps more likely by using Rembrandt than Rothko (but you never know). Otherwise it may work better to allow individuals to hold the stage briefly with work that appeals to them. Ask them to bring along an image that means something to them and to be prepared to say why. There will be disagreements, but these can be used to promote learning about the standpoints of others, given constructive chairmanship.

In one-to-one teaching, it is just as important to allow the learner to suggest examples of art as well as clinical cases. The teacher may have to hold his agenda (and his obsession with Rothko) in check, at least initially.

'Hear, hear!' says Donald.

Whether painters like it or not, many people will find it easier to make their first connection through narrative: stories about people (*see* Chapter 4) and painters (*see* Chapter 5). Paint language (*see* Chapter 7) and meaning (*see* Chapter 6) will probably have to wait.

In Chapter 3, I referred to the work of a group of trainers in Leicester. As a mature group of doctors, we had no difficulty in relating to the connection with 'humanities' and being fellow travellers, with our patients, in the journey through life. This was all very well, but some of us would have been more comfortable with concrete examples of benefit to patients – perhaps an 'art gallery' of diagnosis and treatment.

'I saw a Rembrandt late self-portrait in surgery!' said Dr Strait.
'Well you did, didn't you?' said Dr Susan.
'You mean Mr Choleric,' said Dr Shorts.
'So what's the treatment?' said Dr Strait.

Here is my suggestion – you won't find it in the *BNF*.

- Be fearless.
- Look inside yourself.
- Try to make a connection with the artist and his feelings.
- Find something to help you empathise with the patient.
- Recognise and be recognised as a fellow traveller.

Whilst this feels like the truth to me, I realise that it may be too general for others. So far, at least for the Leicester trainers, specific examples have been hard to come by. Possibly it is because we are all too busy doing our jobs to capture and record such elusive material.

However, two of us[5] have been working on a curriculum for an 'Arts and Medicine' module, based on the sessions about literature, painting and music that have been run by the trainers' group in the last few years. 'Bullet points' were distilled from the discussions we had, and these formed the basis for the curriculum. I have indicated below how they can be related to material in this book.

'Yay!' says Donald. 'At last – lots of lovely bullet points!'
'I must introduce you to Pointillism,' says Liam.

Module overview

This module will focus on an introduction to the use of the 'Arts' in relation to care of patients, and working with colleagues, as people. It will also link with education and professional development. The key areas of the module are:

- the role of the doctor in primary care (Chapter 2)
- the nature of 'Arts' (Chapter 3)
- narrative as an entry to the use of 'Arts' (Chapters 4 and 5)
- feelings and the 'language of the medium' (Chapters 6 and 7)
- reflective practice and professional development (Chapter 8)
- teaching and learning (Chapter 9).

Learning outcomes

As a result of studying this module the student should be able to:

- critically assess the role of the doctor in relation to personal continuing care (Chapter 2)
- critically assess the concept of 'the art of medicine' and the interface between Medicine and the 'Arts' (Chapter 3)

- use narrative as a bridge between Medicine and the 'Arts' (Chapters 4, 5)
- use the 'language of the medium' in relation to feelings of others and self (Chapters 6, 7)
- incorporate use of the 'Arts' into reflective practice, personal development, teaching and learning (Chapters 8, 9).

Detailed curriculum

1   The role of the doctor in relation to personal continuing care:

1.1   patient-centredness
1.2   higher order consulting skills
1.3   the complexity of physical, social, psychological and spiritual presentations
1.4   the concepts of continuity and palliation
1.5   the therapeutic dialogue
1.6   the need for self-awareness
1.7   the need to respect others
1.8   the concept of being a 'fellow traveller'
1.9   work-life balance.

2   The art of medicine and the arts/medicine interface:

2.1   an art with science
2.2   the relevance of 'arts' to the practice of medicine
2.3   the concept of ambiguity
2.4   the concept of 'layers of meaning'
2.5   the relevance of the psychodynamic model
2.6   the relationship between dreams and creativity
2.7   the role of the observer in relation to meaning.

3   Narrative as an entry to the arts:

3.1   relevant social-psychological issues in literature
3.2   accounts of illness and effects on patients and doctors in literature
3.3   patterns of behaviour and illness in literature which relate to current practice
3.4   the effects of mental illness on artists, doctors and patients

3.5 narrative link with other 'arts', such as painting and music
3.6 accounts of behaviour as a link to an appreciation of psychological aspects in 'arts'.

4 Access feelings through the 'language of the medium':

4.1 the nature and degree of 'abstraction', and the link with narrative
4.2 dynamics and emotional drivers
4.3 the complexity of 'meaning'
4.4 relevant examples in poetry, fine art and music
4.5 use of 'arts' in the development of empathy.

5 Use of the arts in reflective practice, professional development, teaching and learning:

5.1 recording relevant experiences in arts and clinical practice
5.2 reflective practice
5.3 reinforcing learning
5.4 professional development
5.5 identifying and addressing future needs
5.6 teaching about arts and clinical practice.

'Are you happy now?' says Liam.
'Yes,' says Donald, 'and I was only winding you up about Rothko!'

References

1 Middleton J (2000) *The Team Guide to Communication.* Radcliffe Medical Press, Oxford.

2 Neighbour R (2004) *The Inner Apprentice: an awareness-centred approach to vocational training for general practice.* Radcliffe Medical Press, Oxford.

3 Thomson L (1998) *Personality Type: an owner's manual.* Shambhala Publications, Boston.

4 Andreas S, Faulkner C and The NLP Comprehensive Team (1996) *NLP: the new technology of achievement.* Nicholas Brealey, London.

5 Middleton J and Drucquer M (2006) Arts and medicine in postgraduate medical education. *Education for Primary Care.* (In press).

Epilogue

'It's no fun getting old,' said Mr. Crepit.

Dr Strait made an effort to look up from the notes. *Self-Portrait 1669 by Rembrandt van Rijn*. He resisted the urge to break eye contact.

'I'm sorry to hear that, Dennis,' he said. 'Can you give me no hope at all?'

A pause, then laughter.

'Well let's just say that it has its moments, doctor!'

'Yes,' said Dr Strait, 'and I want to learn how to concentrate on those moments.'

Index

Page numbers in italic refer to tables.